Hatha Yoga (physical yoga) can bring immense benefits to Western city-dwellers. It teaches the arts of relaxation, of conserving energy, of developing and toning up the whole body. But this book, as well as describing in detail (and with photographs) the physical exercises, also prescribes *mental* exercises for the development of serenity, poise, will-power and inner strength.

Michael Volin, who founded the first yoga school in Sydney, Australia in 1950, has been teaching for thirty years, both in the East and the West. He was first trained in China, where he was born and brought up, and later by Indian and Tibetan teachers. Before he came to Australia he was associated with Indra Devi's yoga school in Shanghai, succeeding her as Director of the school. He is well known in Australia for his television lessons on yoga, as well as through his school in Sydney, and his former pupils are now teaching yoga all over the country.

Nancy Phelan is a Sydney writer, photographer and traveller who has published a novel and two travel books. She has been a serious student of yoga for some years, and was trained as a teacher by Michael Volin. She is now associated with his school and has had a wide experience with pupils of all ages.

All the photographs in this book were taken by *Herman Ilves*. The pupils who posed for them are between the ages of 46 and 73.

YOGA OVER 40

Yoga Over 40
MICHAEL VOLIN AND NANCY PHELAN

SPHERE BOOKS LIMITED LONDON

Copyright © 1965 by Michael Volin and Nancy Phelan

Reprinted by arrangement with Pelham Books Ltd.

First Sphere Books edition, 1967

Reprinted March 1967

Australian Agent: Thomas Nelson (Australia) Limited,
597 Little Collins Street,
Melbourne, Australia.

Canadian Agent: Thomas Nelson and Sons
(Canada) Limited, 81 Curlew Drive,
Don Mills, Ontario.

East African Agent: Thomas Nelson & Sons Limited,
P.O. Box 25012,
Nairobi, Kenya.

Israel Agent: Steimatzky's Agency Ltd.,
Citrus House,
P.O. Box 628,
Tel-Aviv, Israel.

New Zealand Agent: Hodder & Stoughton Limited,
52 Cook Street,
Auckland C.1., New Zealand.

South African Agent: Thomas Nelson & Sons
(South Africa) (Pty) Limited,
Lewis and Marks Building,
65 President Street,
Johannesburg, South Africa.

West African Agent: Thomas Nelson & Sons Limited,
P.O. Box 336,
Apapa, Nigeria.

Printed in Great Britain by
C. Nicholls & Company Ltd.

CONTENTS

Physical and Mental Training

Some of the methods of delaying age included in this book are techniques of *avatara yoga* (see page 18), and have not, to our knowledge, been published before.

ILLUSTRATIONS

Appendix

INTRODUCTION

Many people over forty are confronted with the same physical and mental problems, and need a definite plan for overcoming them.

In any such plan based on yoga, *physical training* would be dedicated to improving the whole condition of the body. This includes:

Correcting weight and figure
Firming and toning-up muscles
Regulating digestive processes
Stimulating circulation of the blood
Limbering-up of joints and spine
Thorough purification of the system

These measures could rejuvenate the body and delay further ageing.

Mental training would include development of inner strength, of a more positive and philosophical attitude to life, overcoming fear of death and achievement of serenity.

*

It is important to understand that there is a difference between yoga as practised by the young and by older students.

Yogis believe that there is no limit to the achievements of one who knows how to combine three powers: power of bodily pose, power of breath, and constructive power of the mind. In yoga over forty the emphasis must be on mental concentration, which is a mighty weapon against ageing when joined with physical exertion.

There must be faith in the constructive power of the mind. A half-hearted attitude is not enough and scepticism negates the benefits of physical practice. Some forty years ago, Coué used the constructive power of the mind very effectively, but his auto-suggestion went only half-way. Yoga's auto-suggestion has the formidable support of physical measures.

Since we live in an age of psycho-analysis and scientific exploration of the mind we know something of its influence on the body; and though the West is still a long way behind the

East in its understanding of this subject, the flood of books on self-improvement, memory training, development of personality, influencing others, mental healing, etc., suggests that the ordinary man and woman is hungry for knowledge and ready to receive it.

Yoga's true message often has its most profound effect on older people. They are more patient, more disposed to listen, and usually life has taught them a true sense of values. It is better to start with a mature, receptive mind and stiff joints, than supple limbs and a shallow, undeveloped mentality, for joints will soon loosen up, but the mind that is not ready may stay closed for years.

*

The nucleus of *Hatha* yoga is the eighty-four traditional *asanas* or bodily positions, but many are too demanding for people past their first youth, particularly if they have not exercised for years. Apart from the poses in the Appendix, we have included nothing that a normal healthy man or woman could not attempt. All contribute to delaying age.

No one is too old for yoga. Even those whose physical condition prevents them from attempting strenuous postures may safely practise relaxation, breathing cycles* and techniques for increasing vital energy. Adjustment of weight and diet, improvement of mental powers and a more positive attitude to life through mental exercises are also within their scope; and for those who are interested, there is the whole field of spiritual development and self-realization. It is with these people in mind that we have included a number of mental and breathing techniques not usually found in popular yoga literature.

*

The old ideas that yoga is "queer" are dying out, but there are still many who think of it as an oriental kind of physical jerks suitable only for the young. Untrained and ignorant people who have set up as teachers to profit from its increasing popularity have contributed to this misconception. True yoga is for anyone and everyone who wants it and age is no barrier.

Though its practice does help in many cases of nervous or

*Breathing is the basis of *Hatha* yoga. In the highest stages of training breathing techniques replace much of the more spectacular physical practices.

physical illness it is not suggested that it is a cure-all. It is mainly a preventive, which, by raising the standard of health, wards off and defeats the first inroads of disease and disability.

This book is concerned with *Hatha* (physical) yoga, but we have included a chapter touching briefly on other paths of yoga, which may serve as a stepping-stone to further reading.

Yoga is not a religion. It is a method of complete development . . . an attitude to life . . . to all creation . . . and its aims are the highest and most noble. All who study it, whatever their personal religion, will find in it something for themselves, and will turn to their own devotions with increased spiritual awareness and understanding.

1

ATTITUDES TO AGE

The western attitude to age

One of the great poems in the English language is Tennyson's *Ulysses* . . . a poem about old age. Its greatness lies not only in the beauty of its words and imagery but in the courage and indomitable spirit it expresses.

After his heroic life of travel and adventure, Ulysses is dissatisfied among people who only "hoard, and sleep, and feed", who think that living is just a matter of continuing to breathe. He knows that twenty lives are not enough for what he wants to do; and though he is old in years he despises the thought of coddling himself while his spirit is still "yearning in desire, To follow knowledge, like a sinking star, beyond the utmost bound of human thought." He must go on sailing "beyond the sunset, and the paths of all the western stars" until he dies; and though he no longer has his former strength, he knows that he is still "strong in will, To strive, to seek, to find and not to yield."

Everyone over the age of forty could take this poem as their inspiration, interpreting it according to their individual capacity. Whether the experiences are physical or in the world of the mind is immaterial; it is the spirit that counts. No matter what age, life should be an endless adventure.

This is not the usual attitude in the West. After years of abusing their bodies, overworking them, filling them with wrong or inadequate foods, with stimulants and tranquillizers, the majority of people over forty have already begun to use the phrase they cling to for the rest of their lives . . . the parrot-cry uttered at every test or challenge, however small . . . "*I'm too old!*" . . . the final excuse for indolence, apathy, self-pity, inefficiency and defeatism.

No one really wants to be Too Old; but only a minority are prepared to exert themselves to delay ageing. They hope, perhaps, that a miracle drug will suddenly solve all their problems, since pills and injections are less trouble than sustained hard work. They rather resemble a man who neglects a good job because he is expecting to win the lottery, who dies in poverty before it ever happens, as these people die, worn out, before the elixir of youth is discovered.

Some years ago a United States magazine asked 400 centenarians what age they would choose to be if they could start life again. The majority said forty-five; not nineteen or thirty but forty-five. It should not be so surprising, for how many people really know how to live in the twenties, even the thirties? The over-forties should be the best age, for a healthy man over forty has a mature mind, an accumulation of experience and a knowledge of life that the young cannot know. He can discriminate between right and wrong; he has stability; clear vision and inner strength; and physically he should be in his prime.

This should be a definite and prolonged stage of life, full of wonderful experiences and achievements . . . a really creative period, crowning the years of development and accumulation, like a long and generous summer when the earth gives back with full hands all that has been sown during the preceding months. We should stay forty-five for thirty years . . . strong, wise, potent, generous, kind, healthy and handsome; but for most people, the forties are accepted as the cancer age, the age of spare tyres, flabby muscles, spectacles, toupees, false teeth, prolapses, impotence, coronary occlusions and hysterectomies.

It is tragic that for most of us this middle period is so short and that it should be regarded as inevitable. We have practically no mature years at all.

Stress, tension, wrong diet, lack of exercise, inadequate rest all help to fill the waiting rooms of doctors and psychiatrists, to increase the number of sudden deaths and nervous breakdowns. This, says western man, is what must be expected over forty.

Yoga's attitude to age

The yogi's attitude to age is quite unlike the western conception. He believes that the physical body does not finish developing until the age of thirty-three (not twenty-one, as we are taught), that even then it may still be remoulded and brought to near-perfection. Fifty-five, which to us is often the beginning of the end, is for the yogi literally the prime of life, the high noon of maturity, while old age, as we know it, need never come at all to one who has learnt the secrets of prolonging youth and life.

A little-known branch of yoga called *Avatara** yoga* is dedica-

Avatara: One who has reached the supreme stage of development, with full power over death and freedom from the law of reincarnation. A fully liberated soul who returns to a physical body to work for the salvation of

ted to this arresting of the ageing process. It embodies the most closely-guarded doctrines of the laws of reincarnation, and includes physical techniques for defying the effects of time. Though there have been very few full *avataras* in the history of mankind, many sages in the closed monasteries of Tibet, India and China study these secret methods of preserving mental and physical powers for extraordinary periods.

The true yogi regards his body as the temple of the living spirit, and his ultimate aim is to liberate that spirit through *yoga* or union with God. For this, the body must be trained into perfect condition and brought under complete control of the mind; and because mental development is much slower than physical, bodily ageing must be delayed, so that maturity of body and mind may be enjoyed together. Like Ulysses, the yogi knows that "life piled on life were all too little", for achieving full development. He must hold back time; and this he knows how to do.

Not all the yogi's techniques are for western students. Some demand complete celibacy, seclusion, austere diet, discipline and immense powers of concentration; but we can adopt his attitude to age, and revise our own ideas as a preliminary to practising some of the more simple methods of holding it at bay.

Everyone over forty should stop and take stock of himself, looking back over the past and forward to the future, dispassionately but constructively. This does not mean brooding on the things you did not do or the opportunities you missed; it means trying to correct past mistakes and to avoid repeating them in the future; it means believing it is never too late to start, and that the future is in one's own hands; it means discarding the conventional attitude to age and dismissing the thought *"Too old"*.

We have all heard of people who looked forward for years to retirement and could not enjoy it when it came because of ill-health and failing powers. Middle-age is the time . . . perhaps the last chance . . . to insure against this tragedy; to make the second half of life a triumphant conclusion to a useful active youth.

---

mankind. His body is immortal. It is said that he makes no footprint and casts no shadow. He does not eat, existing on *prana*. Babaji, the yogi-saint still living in the Himalayas, is an *avatara*, hundreds – perhaps thousands – of years old but with the appearance of a young man.

Every week, newspapers and magazines publish articles on the subject of arresting old age, and some of the world's best brains are engaged in constant research for a means to prolong youth. Remarkable discoveries have been made; but what is perhaps even more remarkable is that the findings of modern geriatricians . . . scientists studying the causes and process of ageing . . . are identical with discoveries made by yogis thousands of years ago.

Scientists tell us that old age is a disease, or a complex of diseases; that the main contributing causes of premature ageing are stress and tension, the presence of foreign germs – however inactive – in the body, lack of exercise, incomplete elimination, which causes chronic poisoning of the system and ultimately the breaking down of certain vital cells. In youth, these cells can repair themselves by division and new growth but with increasing age they lose this power, become clogged with impurities and die. Once dead, some cells cannot be replaced and when, for instance, nerve cells in the brain are thus destroyed, ageing is accelerated.

The ancient yogis knew these facts and evolved techniques for combating them . . . for relaxing tension; for keeping the body healthy and free from infection; for purifying the system by improving elimination . . . even for renewing the cells through breath control and the power of the mind. *They knew that the medium for delaying old age was their own bodies.*

Despite achievements of the drug H3, cellular therapy, synthetic testosterone and transplanting of glands, medical science is now suggesting that research be focused on seeking a method by which the body can continue to repair its own cells, within itself, all through life.

Yoga takes each aspect of ageing in the human body and works on it through diet, rest, purification, breath control, exercises and the constructive power of the mind. It also considers two major factors not sufficiently recognized in the West . . . *the effect of central gravity on the body, and the accumulation and preservation of vital energy.*

Central gravity. The pull of central gravity, which holds us to the earth's surface, is responsible for sagging tissues and muscles, for displaced organs, for loss of youthful buoyancy, for ageing people's increased tendency to sit about or lie down. This downward pull acts upon us all our lives. It is only the conscious will that keeps our bodies upright. The moment we give way . . . as in fainting or in sleep . . . we fall to the ground.

The yogi's main weapon against gravity is the inverted position of the body . . . the shoulderstands and headstands (pages 110–11 and 123), which also increase the supply of arterial blood to head and face, irrigating the brain and stimulating mental processes, feeding the skin and facial tissues, preventing and destroying wrinkles.

Vital energy. Vital energy could be compared to petrol in an automobile. No matter how perfect the condition of mind or body, without vital energy they are useless. When it dies or even flags temporarily we cannot work or enjoy life. Creative powers decline, resulting physically in impotence, and mentally in failure of imagination or the drive needed for expression, so that ideas die in their creators' brains for lack of vital energy to give them birth.

In youth we take our vital energy so much for granted that it never occurs to us it need be guarded and accumulated. Often it is squandered. When, with the passing years, it begins to diminish, we succumb to the pull of gravity; we feel defeated, tired and old.

Prana. In Sanskrit, the ancient language of India, this vital energy, life force or cosmic energy, which is in the air, is known as *prana*. Through the yoga method of improved breathing, more *prana* is taken into the system through the lungs, with the air inhaled, and an extra amount stored for our own use. In this way a tired body can be completely recharged with energy at will, as a battery is charged from the mains. Control of the breath gives control of *prana*, and, it is said, could ultimately lead to control of life itself.

Prana may also be directed to others, with strengthening and healing effects and is the agent whereby many apparently miraculous feats are performed by yogis.

The *pranic* theory must be accepted unconditionally if real success is desired. It is sometimes rejected by conventional materialists, since *prana* has not yet been seen or measured by scientific instruments; fifty years ago such people would have been just as sceptical about vitamins in food.

Physiological and numerical age

Everyone has two ages . . . a numerical age and a physiological age. Numerical age is the number of years since birth, and there

21

is nothing we can do about it; but physiological age, which is manifested by the condition and appearance of the body, can be arrested, even to a certain extent reversed, by ordinary men and women of the West through the serious practice of yoga. There have been many cases of actual rejuvenation in which our students became younger in face and figure, with increased vitality and improved mental faculties, a renewal of virility in men and menstruation in ageing women. It is said that one could prolong the creative part of life by twenty-five years, at the age of seventy looking and feeling no more than forty-five.

These effects are gained through exercises and *asanas* which act on endocrinal glands, the circulation, nervous centres and digestive organs; through learning how to relax and recharge the body; how to improve sleep, combat the forces of gravity, and accumulate and conserve vital energy. The preservation of relative strength (see page 35), and purification through improved elimination, aid the general toning-up of the whole body and mind.

There is nothing mysterious in any of these techniques. They are within the reach of everyone.

Importance of endocrinal glands

We are affected by our glands all through life, but never more so than in middle age. At this time they not only start to show signs of wear and tear in many cases, but in women the whole balance of the glandular system undergoes a profound change with the menopause.

The endocrinal system of ductless glands is made up of the pituitary and pineal glands, both situated in the head; the thyroid and parathyroids, in the throat; the thymus gland, which shrinks with physical maturity, is in the chest; the adrenal glands are set above the kidneys, and the gonads or sex glands, in men, are the testes contained in the testicles, and in women, the ovaries, set low down on each side of the pelvic area.

Each gland or pair of glands has its own vital work to do, but between them all is a subtle relationship, so delicate that if one is out of order, others may be unfavourably affected, with drastic results to mind and body.

The *pituitary* is the master gland, with far-reaching influence on all the others, including the sex glands. The *pineal* helps to keep the endocrinal system in balance and working harmoniously. (The yogi knows it is also the seat of higher faculties . . . of occult powers, clairvoyance, clairaudience and telepathy.) The *thyroid* and *parathyroids* are also key glands, and affect the body's metabolism. Vital energy, increase or loss of weight, the functioning of the sex glands, temperament, mental powers, all come within the thyroid's sphere of influence. If it is over-active the results may be loss of weight, tension, insomnia, palpitations, nerviness and agitation; if it is under-active, increased weight, mental and physical sluggishness, a depressed outlook and apathetic attitude to life can result.

The *adrenal* glands supply us with adrenalin, contributing the energy and drive needed for an active, positive life; while the sex-glands, apart from their importance in the reproductive system, influence the personality, providing feminine warmth and attraction in women and masculine characteristics in men.

Medical researchers tell us that our bodies are provided with a kind of defence system which is called into action in any situation of great pressure or alarm. This system, which works mainly through the adrenal glands, is under the direction of the pituitary. When an emergency is registered in the brain the pituitary sends out a signal, summoning the adrenal glands to action. These glands in turn release into the blood the hormones needed to alert the rest of the body to deal with the danger that threatens.

When an emergency arises, it is not the nature but the *intensity* of the threat that starts the defences working. Serious illness, physical injury, overwhelming grief, acute worry, all have the same power to set off the alarm. After the crisis in accident or illness, or when great anxiety is relieved, the body relaxes its mobilized condition; but as long as the illness is protracted, as long as the worry or grief is sustained, the glands remain in a state of unnatural stress, the adrenals pouring out more and more hormones, till eventually they become exhausted, and illness, even death results.

Yoga's benefits to the endocrinal system are not confined to keeping the glands in good working order. Through relaxing tension, soothing the nerves, developing inner tranquillity and maintaining good health, it helps to reduce the possibility of such destructive processes.

2

PHYSICAL CONDITIONS COMMON IN MIDDLE AGE

It is often in the forties that the harbingers of old age make their first appearance . . . tension, obesity, aches and pains, displaced organs . . . all of which are accepted as a normal part of middle age. Though they are not lethal, they are enough to spoil enjoyment of life, and if left unchecked could lead to more serious maladies. Most of them can be improved by yoga.

Stress and worry

Although these are mental states they are included in this chapter because they often lead to physical illness.

They are the great killers, acting directly through strokes and heart attacks or indirectly through diseases caused by accumulated tension. Because stress and worry are so commonplace they are often regarded as necessary evils, to be endured rather than cured, for doctors will always hand out tranquillizers, and there are temporary escapes, like alcohol and television; but all worry is destructive, even if it does not kill or lead to illness. It is ageing and demoralizing. It is negative because it solves nothing and produces nothing.

Many people are chronic worriers, purely from habit. They lie awake thinking about atom bombs, disasters, financial ruin, sickness, loneliness, old age and other things that may never happen; or they worry because all is going well, like a famous actor who, at the height of his popularity woke regularly in the small hours and panicked about failure and poverty, though he had never been out of work in his life.

These worriers often blame material circumstances, the rush of city life . . . anything rather than admit that the disease lies within themselves. They sometimes become dependent on sedatives and tranquillizers, and they are usually miserable and morose.

Most of them quickly respond to yoga, for when the nerves are relaxed and the glands and circulation are working well, the capacity for futile worrying seems to diminish. Improved health brings a calmer, more easy-going attitude to life. Those who have the perseverence to practice mental exercises have even greater success in freeing themselves of this negative habit.

There are others whose worries are not of their own choosing; but whatever the problem, people trapped in unhappy situations with others dependent on them cannot afford to let their health deteriorate. If they are intelligent they try to analyse their troubles constructively and decide what, if anything, can be done; and if they can do nothing to alter circumstances they must concentrate on getting themselves into the best physical and mental condition for enduring them.

Many such people have turned to yoga. In their dark tunnel it brings a gleam of light, helping them to pull themselves together, first physically, then mentally, and find the inner strength to carry on.

Asanas: General practice, with emphasis on shoulderstand (page 110); headstand (page 123); Triangular Pose (page 111); Fish Pose (page 121); *Savasana* (page 107); and Breathing Cycles (pages 81 and 90); Circulating Life Force (page 84); Pose of a Hero (page 114); Pose of a Child (page 114); Pose of a Frog (page 113).

Mental exercises: Development of Inner strength; I am master of myself; Protective cocoon; and all exercises in Chapter 12 inducing peace, and releasing inner light. Regular meditation on ephemeral nature of most worries. (Read also Chapter 8.)

Hypertension

Stress and worry, for real or imaginary reasons, often lead to hypertension; so do frustrations, constant over-work to the state of exhaustion, too much alcohol and tobacco, not enough exercise, excess weight, and foods that are too fat or too salty. We are also told that reserved natures given to brooding are more susceptible than those who express their emotions freely.

Everyone over forty should have their blood pressure checked regularly; but there is no need to be neurotic about it or to become an invalid if the pressure is too high. The doctor will advise modifying diet, cutting down alcohol and tobacco, and if necessary reducing weight; also taking more rest and mild exercise. Since all these measures are part of its training, yoga has improved many cases of hypertension.

Sometimes high blood-pressure is aggravated by an attitude

to life; a nagging feeling that it has been unfair; of being cheated or exploited; or a driving sense of competition, acquisitiveness, pride, greed or envy. The cause of the trouble can be unbelievably petty . . . other people's possessions, looks, social position, education, financial success . . . but whatever the source, it is the negative thinking evoked that is destructive.

When physical practice is supported by mental exercises it is possible to attain the serenity and inner peace, the philosophical attitude that makes life so much easier to live and enjoy.

Asanas: Prohibited. Headstand. Any inverted pose that brings the blood to the face or head; raised poses which have the same effect, movements swinging downward from the waist; or breathing techniques that build up pressure in the head through retention of breath. *Recommended: Savasana* (pose of complete rest – page 107) peaceful *asanas* such as Fish Pose (page 121); Frog Pose (page 113); Diamond Pose (page 113); Hero Pose (page 114); Lotus Pose (page 113); all the cycles of pacifying breaths (pages 85 and 90).

Mental Exercises: Any or all of the exercises in Chapter 12, especially *Idleness of Mind*. Read also Chapter 4 *Diet*, and Chapter 7 *The different paths of yoga*.

Ulcers

Highly-strung people suffering from ulcers will benefit from regular practice of *Savasana* (page 107), pacifying breathing cycles (page 85–90); Pose of a Frog (page 113); Diamond Pose (page 113); and, if possible, the Lotus (page 113). Strenuous exercises should be avoided; but mental techniques for inducing calmness, inner tranquillity and for relaxing the mind and nerves should be practised. (Chapter 12.)

Heart conditions . . . coronary occlusions

Most of what has been said about hypertension applies to heart conditions. The causes are often the same and the same means may be used to help improve them.

A number of people worry secretly that they have heart trouble, when their symptoms are really caused by nerves or exhaustion or poor physical condition; others are alarmed by old wives' tales, by scraps of information picked up from friends or magazine articles of the Be-your-own-doctor kind. They, too, avoid the doctor for fear of what he will tell them, and this chronic state of anxiety exaggerates their symptoms. When they find there is nothing seriously wrong they usually recover at once.

If you are worried in this way, tell your doctor. Even if you have a heart condition you can do a great deal to help yourself, *with his permission*. Many doctors now recommend yoga for these cases, since regular exercise is part of modern treatment; and relaxation of mind and nerves, an ability to slow down the body and recharge it with energy will speed recovery.

Asanas: In some cases (with doctor's approval) headstand* and shoulderstand (pages 123, 110), all sitting poses (pages 112–116), *savasana* (page 107), spinal massage (page 95), breathing cycles (pages 85 and 90); avoid vigorous and strenuous abdominal or muscular exercises.

Mental: All exercises in Chapter 12. Read also Chapter 3 *Power of the Mind;* Chapter 4 *Diet* and Chapter 7 *The Different paths of yoga.*

Loss of rhythm†

This is a widespread psycho-physical condition in city-dwellers and one that accelerates ageing through its destructive effect on the nervous system, digestion, sleep and physical appearance.

All life is governed by rhythm . . . in the natural world the tides, seasons, night and day, the sun and the moon are some of its familiar manifestations. Human beings also have their rhythm; they cannot live without it. Their bodies are dominated by the rhythmical beating of the heart, the movement of the lungs, the circulation of the blood. Women's bodies are subject to the rhythm of menstruation which, when upset, leads to nervous conditions and physical illnesses: and much has been written to show that ignorance of individual rhythm in intercourse is the chief cause of sexual incompatibility and failure, which also brings nervous and physical disorders, as well as personal tragedies.

In a peaceful, usually rural life, man's individual rhythm can synchronize with the rhythm of nature, producing harmony and

*c.f. The ancient Chinese method of treating heart conditions by suspending upside-down.

†*Rhythm and vibration.* In yoga it is taught that the whole universe is ruled by the law of vibration; that the last, indivisible part of an atom is vibration.

27

tranquillity; but in a great city the constant clash of outer, disturbing vibrations with his inner rhythm, creates discord, tension, neurosis and all the other maladies so familiar to urban people.

Though we cannot all give up our jobs and go and live in the country, yoga can help us to maintain our own rhythm through breathing, relaxing and toning-up the body; and we can further help ourselves by keeping in touch with nature as much as possible – lying on a beach, gardening, walking in the country or by the sea, watching a sunset, a storm, the stars . . . even sitting in a city park looking at pigeons and sparrows . . . taking every opportunity to escape, however briefly, to the eternal, life-giving beauties that are our natural home.

Asanas: Savasana (page 107); Breathing Cycles (pages 82–91); Balancing Poses (pages 117–18); Fish Pose (page 121); Lotus (page 113); Slow movements in Chapter 9; Rocking (page 95); if possible, Raised Poses in Appendix.

Mental Exercises: Concentration; Inner strength; Inner sound; Idleness of mind; creating of Mental *Ashram*; Concentration on breath.

Constipation (See also Chapter 5)

We have already mentioned that constipation is recognized as one of the main causes of ageing.

Bad at any time, it is often a serious problem after middle age, for as the circulation slows down, through lack of exercise, and the muscles lose their tone, through lack of use, the body's eliminative powers deteriorate. Many people who have a bowel movement every day are still partially constipated because evacuation is incomplete.

The bowels should be trained to move *at the same time* every morning, and a cycle of exercises which give internal massage to the abdominal organs must be mastered. There are many other *asanas* and movements which help to correct the condition.

Asanas: Uddiyana (page 124); *Nauli* (page 151); Digestive cycle (page 125); Headstand (page 123); Shoulderstand (page 110); Half-shoulderstand (page 111); Archer (page 120); Spinal Twist (page 120); Cobra (page 121); Locust (page 122); *Yogamudra* (page 115); Head-to-Knee (page 120); Breathing cycles (pages 84–6); *Savasana* (page 107); All forward-stretching cycles (pages 118–19); read also Chapter 4 *Diet* and *fasting*.

Occasionally excess weight is due to some glandular disturbance, but more often it is caused simply by not taking enough exercise and eating too much of the wrong foods.

Very fat people lose much of the joy of life. They look years older than they are; they feel clumsy and tire easily, since it is hard work transporting a great weight about; often suffer from shortness of breath, bronchial weakness and varicose veins; and among women, there can be psychological repercussions, since it is difficult for them to dress well or look attractive. The constant battle of finding clothes to fit, the misery and petty humiliations involved in shopping for them send many women straight to the nearest confectioner or cake-shop for consolation.

It is not only unaesthetic to be too fat in middle age, it is dangerous, for it contributes to diabetes, strokes, coronary occlusions and other heart conditions.

Since this fact has become more widely known there has been an epidemic of dieting and reducing treatments among middle-aged people, often with depressing results. Men and women who have over-indulged in food and physical laziness for years expect to reduce in a matter of days, often subjecting their bodies to severe hardship. If nothing worse, the results are a drawn and lined face, scraggy neck and extreme irritability.

Yoga is a safe way to reduce and control weight, due to its action on the glands. Sometimes the weight is lost quickly; more often it goes slowly, but consistently. There is no need to starve, though obviously fattening foods must be avoided.

The *asanas* and exercises help to keep the body firm while reducing, for when the skin has been stretched to contain large areas of fat over a period of years it loses its elasticity and sags or falls into lines with sudden loss of weight.

If you are too fat, ask your doctor to give you a good reducing diet and keep to it. Watch the calories in your food and make sure that you do not take in more than you can use up. Remember that you need less food as you get older. Checking the weight every day on bathroom scales helps to strengthen morale and determination. Exercise regularly in the open air. Try to use the car less and walk more. Garden, if you can, swim or play squash or tennis; but of all exercise, yoga is the most rewarding, bringing not only a painless reduction in weight but improvement in health, increase in energy and *joie de vivre*. (This subject is dealt with more fully in Chapter 4 *Diet*.)

Asanas: Shoulderstand (page 110); Headstand (page 123); Plough (page 119); Head-to-Knee (page 120); Spinal Twist (page 120); Archer (page 120); Sideways Swing (page 121); *Uddiyana* (page 124); Arch Gesture (page 118); Lotus (page 113); Exercises in Chapter 9 (page 92).

Stiffness of joints

This is a typical sign of premature ageing and one that should never be allowed to develop, for apart from arthritic conditions, stiff joints come from lack of exercise.

Our bodies were meant for movement, for walking, running, climbing, bending . . . not for sitting all day at a desk and driving everywhere by car. We are told that we started as legless creatures crawling out of the water. Are we to end up the same way . . . our legs atrophied for want of use? Though modern legs are longer and better-looking than, for instance, those of our medieval ancestors, they are not so strong or so well-developed.

Our children are literally forgetting how to walk. Most of them do not even have the excellent exercise of going up and down stairs, since so many modern houses are built on one level. They are driven to school and brought home by car or bus. At weekends no one goes for walks; they go for drives. It is quite common for young people to complain that their legs ache if they walk any distance at all.

Men and women who are now over forty may have done more walking in their youth than their children do, but it does not mean they are in good condition. Busy housewives who are always on their feet are only partially exercising their bodies (and often in fatiguing circumstances) and even people who still participate in active sport only use certain sets of muscles.

The best way to fight stiffness and keep the joints mobile is to give them regular exercise, preferably at the same time every day. Yoga, which works systematically on every part of the body, is the most satisfactory method for achieving an all-over loosening-up, especially for city dwellers, who are usually in such a chronic state of hurry that they cannot spare the time to walk one block. After a day standing at a stove or behind a counter, sitting at a desk or driving a bus, the stiff body may be gently limbered up, the spine made flexible, and fresh arterial blood sent to the roots of the spinal nerves.

Asanas and exercises: All exercises in Chapter 9; Stretching cycle (page 118); Cobra (page 121); Locust (page 122); Plough (page 119); Spinal Twist (page 120); Archer (page 120); Lotus (page 113); Head-to-Knee, sitting and standing (pages 118–20); Diamond Pose (page 113); Frog Pose (page 113); Hero Pose (page 114).

Arthritis and rheumatism

In the past, victims of these complaints were advised to avoid movement, were even kept in bed, so that they became completely crippled. Many doctors now recommend constant exercise to prevent immobilization, and often suggest yoga.

Though no claims are made that it cures these conditions, yoga does delay their progress by keeping the joints movable, and by raising the general standard of health, helps the body to hold the disease at bay.

Through their action on the adrenal glands, certain *asanas* have a direct effect on rheumatism. These are Cobra (page 121); Spinal Twist (page 120); Bow (Appendix); Lotus position (page 113); Head-to-knee, sitting and standing (pages 118 and 120); and Arch gesture (page 118); for rheumatism and arthritis generally, practise all possible *asanas* and exercises.

Sciatica

The Spinal Twist (page 120); Head-to-knee pose, sitting and standing (pages 118 and 120); and Arch gesture (page 118); are all recommended for the relief of sciatica.

Backache

This is one of the most common complaints of modern life and is responsible for thousands of lost working-hours all over the world.

Many pupils with different back complaints have passed through Michael Volin's yoga school – most of them sent by doctors – and the vast majority have benefited, for since yoga puts such emphasis on the development of a healthy spine and back there are many exercises and *asanas* expressly designed for that area. Every case of backache must be regarded as individual, but in general, treatment lies in strengthening and limbering-up the spine, and invigorating the roots of the spinal nerves.

Asanas: Inverted poses (pages 109–12); Cobra (page 122); Locust (page 122); Twist (page 120); Archer (page 120); Stretching cycles (page 118); Limbering-up exercises and spinal exercises and massage (rocking) (page 95); in Chapter 9; *Savasana* (page 107).

Mental Exercises: Concentration on Breath; breathing away pain; directing *prana* to spine.

Insomnia

Since sleep and insomnia are discussed at some length in Chapter 5 it is only necessary to mention here that there are various physical impediments to good sleep which can be eliminated; that it is possible to learn how to improve the quality of sleep, and to overcome dependence on sleeping pills through certain yoga exercises and *asanas*.

Asanas: Headstand (page 123); Pose of Tranquillity (page 111); Spinal massage (rocking) (page 95); quiet breathing cycles (page 90); *Savasana* (page 109).

Mental Exercises: Idleness of mind; Blankness of mind; Mental Ashram; all exercises for relaxing and soothing the mind.

Prolapse of the uterus

Prolapse, which is fairly common in middle-aged women, occurs when through muscular weakness or excessive child-bearing the uterus is affected by the pull of central gravity and becomes displaced. Surgery was the usual treatment, but it is a painful operation that most women would prefer to avoid, and an increasing number of doctors now recommend exercise.

The most important and powerful *asanas* for this complaint are the Headstand (page 123) and Shoulderstands (page 110); *aswini mudra* (page 116); *Prohibition:* Strenuous raised poses (pages 124 and 152) which tone up and strengthen the abdominal muscles.

Enlargement of the prostate gland

This most unpleasant condition, which often affects older men, may, with the doctor's approval, be helped by *aswini mudra* (page 116); Arch Gesture (page 118); Stretching Cycle (pages 118–20); *Vajroli mudra* (page 116); Frog Pose (page 113) and massage (given on page 34).

Loss of vital energy

This is discussed in Chapter 1, page 21, and in Chapter 8 (Breathing) methods of accumulating and conserving life force are described.

Everyone over forty should take the subject very seriously and make genuine efforts to increase and preserve their vital energy as a safeguard against an unhappy old age.

Asanas: Shoulderstand (page 110); Headstand (page 123); Fish Pose (page 121); Circulating life force (page 84); Head-to-knee (page 120); Knees-to-stomach (page 123); *Vajroli mudra* (page 116).

Varicose veins

Tight shoes, pregnancy, excess weight, too much sitting about, occupations involving too much standing, not enough walking, all contribute to and aggravate varicose veins. Regular practice of the inverted *asanas* will always improve, sometimes completely cure the condition, and exercises for stimulating the circulation should also be included (Chapter 9).

Any pose that puts undue pressure on the legs, such as sitting back on the heels, or cuts off the circulation in that area, such as the Lotus or Half-Lotus pose, should not be practised.

People with varicose veins who spend all day at a desk or table should stand up and move about from time to time so the circulation does not become blocked. They should also sit well back on the chair so that the weight of the body is evenly distributed and not concentrated on the thighs. Pressing the thighs against the hard edge of a seat for hours at a time could cause a thrombosis (clot) in a weakened vein; and sitting with the legs crossed, so that one thigh weighs heavily on the other, could bring the same result. A footstool will help to relieve pressure in sitting.

Asanas: Headstand (page 128); all inverted poses (pages 109–12); circulation exercises in Chapter 9 (page 93).

Haemorrhoids

Since these are a form of varicose veins, which are aggravated by constipation, they will be improved by the *asanas* recommended for both these conditions . . . stomach contractions (pages 124 and 151); inverted poses (pages 109–12) and general toning-up movements. Exercises for the circulation should also be added, and *aswini mudra* (page 116) which has a direct effect on the area concerned. Also practise walking on the buttocks (Chapter 9, page 100) and the following movement for massage: Sit with knees bent and spread apart and the soles of the feet together. Holding the ankles, rock the body from side to side, gently massaging the rectum.

Conditions in feet and ankles

Swelling in feet and ankles should be reported to a doctor, since it could be a symptom of heart or kidney disease. It is usually neither, in which case all the inverted poses are recommended.

For *cold feet*, the circulation exercises in Chapter 9 should be practised, night and morning; and Triangular Pose (page 111) just before bedtime.

Many women with good figures and pretty faces have hideous crooked feet, covered with corns. Tight shoes are usually the cause of these deformities and in the last few years pointed toes have completed any damage started in youth.

It is unrealistic to ask women to give up wearing elegant shoes, but after the age of forty-five some sort of compromise must be worked out if the feet are not to become a liability.

Try to wear high heels only for special occasions, not for walking round the town or standing all day behind a counter. Go barefoot as much as possible . . . at the beach, in the country, in the garden. Take off your shoes as soon as you come into the house. Bathe, oil and massage the feet whenever they are tired and take the weight off them as often as possible by practising the inverted poses.

Remember also that cheap shoes are a false economy all round and shoes that are too tight are ruinous. Reduce, if overweight, and strengthen feet and ankles by foot exercises (pages 94 and 103); Eagle Pose (page 117); Lotus Pose (page 113); Hero Pose (page 114).

Deterioration of skin, tissues and muscles

When the circulation slows down, with increasing age and decreasing activity, one of the first parts of the body affected is the face. Starved of blood, it grows wrinkled and lined, while the tissues, fighting a losing battle against the pull of gravity, begin to sag, giving a drawn and haggard appearance.

There is a set of yogic exercises which, if practised regularly, will help to keep the facial muscles firm; and all positions that bring blood to the face will feed the tissues, tone up the skin and stave off wrinkles.

Proper breathing is essential for a glowing healthy skin, and diet, sleep and relaxation are also important. Constipation dulls the complexion; malnutrition causes sagging and wrinkles; overeating brings blotches and blemishes. Lack of sleep shows as pouches under the eyes, and tension as lines and an ageing expression.

Asanas and exercises: Facial exercises in Chapter 11; Breathing cycles (pages 85–91); Half-shoulderstand (page 111); Headstand (page 123); Head of a cow pose (page 116); Knee-to-stomach (page 123); *yoga-mudra* (page 115). All forward-stretching movements (pages 118–20) and any exercise that involves swinging downward from the waist . . . Chapter 9. If possible, the raised poses in the Appendix. (*All these exercises and asanas are forbidden where there is high blood pressure.*)

Exercises for firming the muscles and sculpturing the body are given in Chapter 9. Read also Chapter 4, *Diet*; Chapter 5, *Care of the skin.*

Loss of relative strength

Relative strength could be described as the strength of the muscles in relation to the weight of the body. When we are young our relative strength is high. A healthy youth can pull himself up fifteen or twenty times, lifting the whole weight of his body without effort. This wonderful lightness usually disappears with age, even if the body does not become overweight, and most middle-aged people move heavily, without buoyancy.

The yogis believe that we should always be able to lift our own weight without effort, and that we should stay light and buoyant all our lives. These qualities are preserved through the Raised Poses (see Appendix), in which the body is elevated and supported on the hands. Though these positions are rather strenuous for older people, they are not always beyond their capacity, providing there is no physical reason to forbid them.

These *asanas* are also rejuvenators because they bring extra blood to the facial skin and tissues. They are stimulating and invigorating and contribute greatly to the development or recovery of self-confidence, which so often fails in middle age.

3

MENTAL CONDITIONS COMMON IN MIDDLE AGE

Depression

Though we know that the mind can work on the body to cause illness, we sometimes forget that the body also works on the mind, and that a low physical condition could cause all sorts of mental disturbances.

Many of the negative states of mind common in middle-age originate in this way, for they are a manifestation of decreasing vitality.

Sometimes in the forties and fifties there comes a curious sensation of having stepped outside life. People suddenly feel that they are no longer moving along in the current but are stranded on the banks, watching. They see themselves in relation to their setting with a devastating clarity, which is often coloured by the state of mind or health. Life no longer has any purpose or meaning. They feel profound disillusionment, despondency and despair. In extreme cases they have turned to suicide.

However desolating this experience, it must be recognized for what it is: a symptom of weakness, as a sore throat or a temperature are symptoms of physical illness. The realization of this fact is half the battle in regaining a proper perspective on life; and once you know that the condition can be remedied by proper treatment it should be easier to endure it when it comes, and work to discourage its recurrence.

Even while you are still subject to these moods . . . for that is all they are . . . you could turn them into a positive experience by using them to take stock of yourself; to look at your life objectively and decide where you will go from here . . . not in the material sense but in your personal development. The mental techniques in Chapter 12 will help to develop inner strength and a more courageous and constructive attitude to life, but improvement of the physical condition is also essential.

Vital energy must be increased and preserved, the nerves relaxed, sleep improved and glands and vital centres toned up. It may also be necessary to adjust the diet, for there could be a vitamin deficiency.

Usually, a higher state of physical well-being means less mental depression, but if after all these measures have been taken you still feel life has no purpose, try taking your mind off yourself. If you have no dependents or friends, go to a hospital, a psychiatric clinic, a rehabilitation centre, a school for spastic or subnormal children and see how people with real troubles manage to live. Better still, do something to help them. In this way you will also help yourself.

Asanas recommended: Savasana (page 107); Breathing cycles (pages 85–91); Headstand (page 123); Inverted poses (pages 109–12); Fish (page 121); Spinal twist (page 120); Cobra (page 121); Forward-stretching (pages 118–20); Lotus (page 113); *vajrolimudra* (page 116).

Mental exercises: Sorting seeds of thought; Inner strength; I am master of myself; I am Stronger than Fear; Read Chapters 7 and 12.

Lack of confidence

Lack of confidence in middle-age also derives from diminishing vital energy. Most of us know the exhaustion that comes after strain and exertion and goes after a good night's sleep; but sometimes in middle-age it becomes chronic. We are always tired; we cannot cope; we start to talk of being too old. We hesitate, afraid of risk, afraid of failure. First the spirit, then the flesh begins to falter. Old age, with all its traditional miseries, is accepted.

Though material possessions are an undoubted comfort to ageing people they do not solve everything. Far more important are an ability to revalue time, to adapt to changes within oneself, to accumulate vital energy and maintain a philosophic attitude towards whatever life brings. No one who has these assets is likely to lose confidence, for there is little that can shake him.

Confidence is often confused with aggressiveness, though one is based on inner strength and certainty and the other usually springs from a deep sense of uncertainty, even inferiority. Aggressiveness is no real friend to a man and it is well if he loses it; but true confidence, which is quiet and serene, is a lasting benefit. It communicates itself to others, commanding respect, and supports those who possess it.

Asanas and exercises: Savasana (page 107); Vital energy recharging (pages 84–7); Breathing cycles (pages 82–5); Balancing poses (pages 117–18); Shoulderstand (page 110); Headstand (page

123); if possible, the Raised Poses in the Appendix. Lotus pose (page 113); Pose of a Hero (page 114); Cobra (page 121); Spinal twist (page 120); *Vajroli mudra* (page 116); Angular pose (page 117).

Mental exercises: I am stronger than fear; Inner strength; I am master of myself.

Failing memory and powers of concentration

The headstand is the most important *asana* for these conditions because it stimulates the brain, but all general practice should be carried out to tone up glands, organs and circulation. Improved physical health strengthens mental powers.

Read Chapter 12 (Mental training) carefully, for all the exercises given there are important, especially Stillness of the Mind, Concentration, Developing of Mind's Eye, Development of Will Power, Creating of the Flower and all exercises concerned with concentration.

Fear

Many people are dominated by fear of some sort . . . fear of poverty, of illness, of loneliness, fear of the unknown, of war, of world destruction . . . of death . . . or in its worst and most dangerous form, fear itself . . . the fear of fear.

It is absurd and humiliating that man, who has achieved such triumphs in the fields of art, science and technology, should be enslaved by something so primitive and negative as this ancient inheritance from our earliest ancestors. It is worth making every effort to be free of it, to be able to regard life as a challenge, not a threat.

A generally timid attitude often comes from anaemia, poor nerves and low vitality; and morbid obsessions, sombre forebodings can originate in the digestive system. (Chekhov, the famous writer, who was also a doctor, once advised a patient who complained of depression: "If you give up eating pork and drinking vodka before retiring, all your depression will be gone".)

When the body is strengthened, conditioned and calmed, much of this distressing state of mind disappears; and mental training brings more confidence and courage to face life.

Asanas: Headstand (page 123); Shoulderstand (page 110); Triangular Pose (page 111); *Savasana* (page 107); Breathing (pages 85–91); Cobra (page 121); Locust (page 122); Spinal Twist (page 120); Lotus (page 113); Balancing poses (page 117); Pose of a Hero (page 114); *Vajroli mudra* (page 116); *Mental Exercises:* Inner strength; Seven Fears; I am Master of Myself; Read Chapters 7 and 12.

Retirement

When active people are obliged to slow down they often become aimless, discontented and depressed. Every day, men are retiring from their jobs and starting on a downward path of degeneration because of boredom and the feeling that they are no longer needed. Doctors say that this loss of purpose is one reason why men die earlier than women. Stress is bad, but complete lack of any kind of stress is also destructive. After a lifetime of battle most men cannot support the anticlimax of retirement.

At first a man may be buoyed up by the farewell parties and presentations, the idea of a long holiday; then he starts to miss the familiar routine, the office staff, the demands of work. He forgets how much he hated the routine, that he did not really like his office companions, that the frustrations of his job nearly brought him a nervous breakdown. He sinks into melancholy and self-pity. He drives his wife to distraction. He doesn't know what to do with himself. He never cared for reading or gardening – he always depended on others – but now he is so gloomy and full of complaints that people avoid him. He sits alone watching television, unable to understand why he no longer finds it amusing or satisfying, or goes on errands for his wife. His movements lose all buoyancy and become shuffling; his mind degenerates. He sees nothing but his own unhappiness. He is old.

The commonplace tragedy of looking forward to retirement and being physically unable to enjoy it when it comes is nothing to the fate of people condemned to a slow decline with no inner resources to sustain them.

Physical yoga could help many to prolong their active lives, but even where some disability prevents this there are still adventures of the mind and spirit, for those who are willing to explore them, to draw apart a little, to watch and think. The man who has not waited till old age to make these discoveries finds no terrors in a physical slowing-down, and has the advantage over the man who has always lived on the surface; but, it is better to come to them late than never come at all. Eventually we all reach the age when our focus changes, turning inwards upon ourselves. If there is nothing for us to find there, life loses purpose, the mind becomes full of discontent.

Men and women who cannot accept this, who cannot bear to leave the party, dreading silence and solitude, always show their age; not perhaps in lines and grey hair, but in their restless unhappy eyes, their brittle voices and their emptiness of mind and life.

A famous wise man once said, "The most fascinating journey I ever made was the journey into myself." It is an endless journey, full of discovery.

Mental exercises: Sorting Seeds of Thoughts; regular meditation and all mental exercises in Chapter 12.

Yoga and the power of the mind in illness

When the mind works morbidly on the body it can wreak terrible havoc. Emotional disturbances, mental shock or exhaustion can all manifest themselves as symptoms of illness in physically healthy people . . . as false cardiac conditions, ulcers, skin rashes, sinus troubles or asthma. Paralysis of speech or body have resulted from acute mental stress, and extreme states of hysteria can produce open sores or ulcers, or agonizing pains which are actually felt by the sufferer, and which occur regularly in organically sound bodies. Yet the mind is also the greatest healer of all. In serious illness, when medical skill has been exhausted, it is the only power that can effect the final cure, for if the patient's mind does not bid him fight and live he dies; and in defiance of all medical opinion, it can bring about miraculous recoveries.

The crutches and leg-irons hanging in the Grotto at Lourdes, the wax replicas and plaster casts in churches all over the world testify to these healing powers. Faith can move mountains; and whether it is the sufferer himself or the Virgin Mary or St. Bernadette who performs the miracle, the medium through which it is done is the patient's own mind. These devout people are cured not as a reward for their devotions, but because of the power of their faith; because of the extraordinary concentration of all their strength and energies into the desire to be healed and the belief that they will be healed.

Hundreds of people are helping to cure themselves of various illnesses through yoga and the power of their own minds. The most common cures are in asthma, migraine, hypertensions, insomnia, indigestion, "nerves", varicose veins, sinus troubles, addiction to tranquillizers, sleeping pills and smoking; but there are other, more complex conditions which have been relieved. A woman writes that she has recovered from a rare blood condition; another, that yoga cured her of angina pectoris; a man whose nerves were "torn to pieces" with dermatitis and who had received no relief from specialists, believes that yoga not only cured the skin complaint but restored his nerves and powers of sleep; a man of 72, whose bronchial trouble was said to be incurable, since it was nervous in origin, claims he has been cured and enabled to return to work; and victims of strokes and polio have recovered the use of their limbs by re-educating them through yoga.

These men and women are of every age and from completely different walks of life, yet all have one quality in common. *They wanted to be helped, and they believed that yoga could help them.* Without this belief, without this powerful co-operation of the mind, the cures might not have been effected.

Almost every week, patients whose maladies are mental in origin are sent to us by doctors, and some psychiatric hospitals now include yoga in their therapy.

At the moment of writing this book, a pupil, sent by her doctor at a psychiatric centre, is making determined efforts to save herself from a mysterious malady which has three times sent her into mental hospital. Specialists can only tell her it is "nerves"; that they can do nothing, though she endures agonizing pain. She says that yoga is her only salvation. If she practises each night the pain is relieved and she can sleep without drugs; if she does not practise the pain returns. Although she still suffers intensely, her general health has already improved and if she does recover it will be because of her own will-power and her belief in the healing power of yoga.

Another pupil in her early forties was told some years ago by a doctor that she would "be on tranquillizers for the rest of her life". Her health was deteriorating and having tried every other cure, her vicar suggested yoga.

She has intense faith; she believes she is going to be cured and now that her health is better, has already given up her thrice-daily dose of sedation. She is trying now to sleep at night without drugs, and eventually she will succeed.

These two modern women are following the ancient yoga teaching that the power of bodily pose, power of breath and constructive power of the mind, *when used together*, can overcome all obstacles.

4

DIET, FASTING, ALCOHOL, TOBACCO

Most middle-aged people have had the experience of suddenly meeting an old school friend after many years and finding them unrecognizable. Sometimes the change has been wrought by hardship, illness or suffering, but quite often it is the result of prosperity. In these strangers with their florid complexions, bald heads, gross stomachs and thick necks we seek in vain for the slim young girl or handsome youth we knew.

The sad thing is that it need not have happened. These men and women are the victims of their own ignorance and lack of discipline.

The story is usually the same. In youth they were active and fond of sport. Their appetites were good; they ate anything and everything and their stomachs digested whatever they consumed. With increasing age and prosperity, physical activity diminished, sport was given up, they drove instead of walking; but the eating went on, bigger and better than ever. The slim girls, now married and mothers of families, went to coffee parties, tea parties, bridge parties, all occasions for eating fattening foods; they cooked for their husbands and children, tasted as they cooked, cleaned up their children's left-over puddings and cakes. They ate at the cinema and while watching television; they drank more alcohol. They put on weight, at first with resentment, then with resignation, finally with apathy. They took ever larger sizes in clothes, gave up active games because they were short of breath, even stopped going to the beach because they looked ugly in swimming costume, sat about more and often ate increasingly as consolation for their discontent.

The men, the active swimmers and surfers, the footballers, cricketers, athletes and rowers gradually became watchers rather than participators. They married. They dropped out of sporting circles, stayed at home with their families or took them for picnics (in the car). Some might do a little gardening . . . slowly following a power mower across the lawn; or at the beach they might briefly dip into the sea between sunbaking; but for the most part, week-ends would be spent entertaining friends with dinner parties, Sunday brunches, barbecues and beer, drinks on the terrace.

On weekdays there were business lunches to fill them up at mid-day a few drinks after work and perhaps a few more at home; then a substantial dinner, followed by television and TV snacks.

The conclusion is logical. Less exercise + more eating = excess weight, with all its attendant maladies.

It is ironic that by the time most of us can afford to indulge in rich living our bodies cannot accept it. We cannot take liberties with middle-aged digestions which, if abused in youth, are starting to show signs of wear and tear. In any case we need less food as we get older. With decreased physical activity we burn it up less quickly and it goes to fat; and every day we are warned of the dangers of excess weight. We are told that it puts a strain on the heart, that it contributes to coronary occlusions (which are less common in countries where the population is not so well fed), that animal fats build up cholesterol in the arteries and lead to strokes.

The remedy lies in regular exercise and suitable diet . . . well-balanced, health-giving meals . . . not in fads and freak diets, which are as bad as over-eating. There is nothing so trying as a health-food crank who fusses endlessly about his diet, cannot eat this and that, constantly switches to new and wonderful – and usually unpalatable – discoveries. Most freak diets are useless for keeping the weight down. Some advocate eating nothing but meat; others recommend milk and bananas. One suggests eating only one meal a day, another is mainly composed of eggs; some are entirely deficient in nourishment, promoting only indigestion, haggard faces and bad temper.

Every city now has slimming parlours or health studios where weight is taken off by sometimes drastic and brutal methods. Steaming, vibrator belts, violent exercise and starvation diets are not only foolish but dangerous for many middle-aged people; and usually the first large meal puts on most of the weight so painfully removed. Dehydrating diets are completely unrealistic, apart from their bad effect on the kidneys, for the weight increases again with the first cup of liquid taken; and the lined, sagging necks and faces that result destroy any illusion of youth given by the hard-won slender body.

Most middle-aged women know that they cannot afford to get too thin too suddenly, but men sometimes overlook this fact. A healthy man in his fifties, alarmed by talk of coronary occlusions, recently embarked on a drastic diet, accompanied by steam-baths, and lost several stone in a very short time. From the back he looked much younger; but his face, which had been firm and fresh, suddenly fell into hundreds of tiny lines, adding years to his age.

If you are too fat you must reduce carefully and slowly, through exercise and diet. At one time there was a belief that exercise had no influence on weight; but this idea has now been discarded. Tests have shown that men do not gain weight when they exercise but put it on when they stop, although eating exactly the same food.

Yoga *asanas*, through their effect on the glands, not only reduce the weight and keep it down, but redistribute it over the body, bringing greatly improved proportions, while at the same time keeping muscles and tissues firm and preventing the unsightly flabbiness that usually accompanies loss of weight. Even yoga exercises must be supplemented by proper diet. This does not mean renunciation of all normal food, as some people imagine, but it does mean giving up all those things which you should never have been eating in the first place.

All diets are improved by eliminating white bread, white sugar, sweets, artificially flavoured drinks, alcohol, chocolates, cakes, biscuits, pastries and fried foods, which are all rich in calories, low nutritionally, mostly indigestible and bad for the teeth. On the other hand, butter, and the much-abused potato are not only valuable nourishment but contain less calories than many other foods (one 3-oz. potato has 72 calories; one slice of chocolate cake has 215; a dessertspoon of butter has 53 calories, and a 2-oz. glass of brandy or gin contains 110).

We must have sugar to give us energy, but we should get it from honey, from dried or fresh fruits, which also purify the blood. A dessertspoon of honey taken at breakfast each morning destroys a craving for sweets and chocolates, yet it contains only 32 calories as against 18 in every teaspoon of sugar. Those who take sugar in tea and coffee, and who eat sweets and cakes, must consume a great many teaspoons during the day. Try to use honey for sweetening instead.

For those who are underweight, yoga suggests the following remedy: practise the Candle position (page 110) as often and for as long as possible (to invigorate the thyroid and metabolic processes); then drink warm goat's milk, immediately afterwards. Practise the body-building exercises in Chapter 9, regularly, without fail.

The true yoga diet, which is mainly lacto-vegetarian, may not be suitable for an active businessman living in a northern European city, but we can learn much from the yogi's knowledge of foods and their effects on the body. The three main dietary principles, which are especially important for older people, are *selectivity, moderation, and mastication*. Select only good and nourishing food; do not overeat or take anything to excess; and chew thoroughly, remembering that mastication is the first stage in the digestive process and if it is rushed or skimped the result will be dyspepsia, no matter how excellent the diet.

Moderation also means common sense, not going to extremes. You will improve health as well as figure by avoiding artificial or over-processed food, by increasing your intake of vegetables and fruit, eating them raw whenever possible; by sometimes substituting eggs and cheese for meat. It is not necessary to become entirely vegetarian, but meat once a day is more than enough, especially after forty. Fish or chicken could be taken instead of the heavier, richer beef or pork.

Meat (or flesh) is not included in a real yogi's diet, partly because it involves taking life, and partly for reasons of purification.

There is an idea that vegetarian diet makes people weak; yet there have been many excellent vegetarian athletes and swimmers; and no one would suggest that the vegetarian gorilla is a weakling.

Fresh fruit at breakfast, fruit juices, *fresh and interesting* salads . . . not gloomy unimaginative mixtures of tinned peas, wilted lettuce and tomato . . . should all be eaten every day. In hot weather, cold meals are welcome, but salads should not be abandoned in winter, while ingredients are available. A fresh crisp green salad of some kind . . . lettuce, endive, raw cabbage . . . should follow the main course. An oil and lemon-juice dressing will give it more character.

Yoghurt is an excellent food and rewards overcoming any initial dislike. It is nourishing, easily digested and highly beneficial to the alimentary system. For a summer lunch, fruit salad of whatever is available with yoghurt (instead of cream), honey (instead of sugar) and roasted almonds is delicious, slimming and sustaining; while yoghurt with honey or fruit makes a light and admirable breakfast, not only for inactive people but for those who are in the habit of rushing off immediately after meals.

This, of course, is a very bad practice and should be corrected.

All meals should be eaten in peace, especially breakfast, which can set the mood for the whole day. A large meal of bacon and eggs, bolted down under pressure, soon develops into a hard lump or a feeling of nausea or acidity or some other familiar and disagreeable symptom. Heavy meals late at night are also unwise and are a common cause of insomnia.

There is no doubt that the most sensible western meal arrangements are those in countries like France and Italy, where breakfast is light, the main meal is at midday, with plenty of time for eating and digesting, and even having a siesta, and a lighter meal follows in the evening.

Liquids

The body must be kept supplied with adequate fluid. Water is the best drink of all . . . cheap, purifying and non-fattening, unless gulped down with bread or heavy food.

Fresh (not tinned) fruit or vegetable juices are also excellent, and everyone who possibly can should buy a juice extractor so that a regular supply of fresh juice is available. With this simple machine all kinds of fruits, or vegetables, may be squeezed together. Pineapple, grapes, peaches, oranges and passionfruit, or other combinations are delicious; while fresh grape juice is not only good to taste but has healing powers.

The juice should be made as it is needed, not stored in the refrigerator.

In summer, cultured buttermilk is a very good drink, nourishing and not fattening; and milk is a food as well as a drink. Many old people live almost entirely on milk, retaining clear eyes and complexions and healthy digestive systems. Drink it slowly, without gulping, as if "chewing" each mouthful.

Since everyone cannot take milk, or may be forbidden it because of weight, an excellent substitute is a drink made with 50 per cent yoghurt and 50 per cent water, beaten up like a milkshake, with a pinch of salt. This drink is popular in Turkey, where it is known as *ayran*, and one can work and travel long distances on little else, without hunger or fatigue, especially in hot weather.

Alcohol

Alcohol, with its high sugar content, is a great fattener; it is also, of course, an artificial stimulant which can become second nature when too frequently taken. In excess, it ruins complexion, nerves and digestion, for it is a form of poisoning (hence the word intoxication). High blood-pressure, cirrhosis of the liver, mental degeneration are a few of the maladies it can produce, not to mention the complete destruction of willpower and character.

No serious yoga student would so destroy his health or body; yet there are many social occasions in western life when it is difficult to avoid alcohol entirely. If you feel you are strong enough to take a drink without going any further, there is little harm in doing so occasionally, but if you know yourself to be incapable of calling a halt, refuse it altogether. No really mature person can be shamed or blackmailed into drinking if they decide against it, and people who insist on forcing their guests to drink out of stupidity or false hospitality are best avoided.

In middle-age and after, it is important to cut down the consumption of hard liquor, and better still to give it up altogether. Wine, which contains less alcohol and less calories, is not so harmful, *in moderation*, since it is made from grapes that have ripened in the sun, absorbing its life-giving properties, its vitamin D. In Italy, where it is considered as much a part of the poor man's diet as bread, spirits are rarely drunk and drunkenness is almost unknown.

The rule of selectivity and moderation should be applied to wine as to food. Drink only good wine, and never to excess.

Tobacco

There has now been so much publicity given to the direct connection between smoking and lung cancer that it seems hardly necessary to raise the subject here; yet despite all the campaigning there are still many people who continue to smoke heavily.

For any yoga student to smoke is a contradiction in terms and a complete waste of effort. It is hardly worth practising breathing exercises if you follow them by inhaling lung-fulls of poisonous nicotine. As an illustration of the degree of saturation reached by a smoker's system, a student who had formerly been a heavy smoker for years but who had broken the habit, reported that even six months after his last cigarette his skin still sweated nicotine when he took a sauna bath.

Apart from lung cancer, heavy smoking contributes to chronic bronchitis, emphysema (degeneration of elastic lung tissue) and coronary disease. Through its action in the bloodstream it affects digestion, the condition of the skin and particularly the nervous system. Like any narcotic, it feeds upon itself and its victim, who grows increasingly dependent on it. It lifts, then lets down; it soothes the nerves, then irritates them into an urgent craving for more. Its apparent benefits are in fact destructive, for the stimulation is false, dragged from an already weakened reserve and never replenished. Eventually the whole store of vital energy is gone and premature decay begins.

Smoking is thus in direct opposition to yoga training, which concentrates on methods of increasing and building up permanent stocks of vital energy, through breath control. Yoga often causes an unconscious inhibition of smoking, for with an acquired ability to relax, the nerves are less in need of artificial soothing; while for those who really want to break the habit the practice of self-hypnosis is advised. Many of our students have cured themselves in this way.

Start with meditation on the subject of smoking.

1. Sit cross-legged in a secluded place, preferably in the open, and establish deep breathing.* Enjoy every moment of it, concentrating on the thought of the purity of the air, the pleasure of inhaling it, the delicate tissues of the lungs and how easily they can be damaged.

2. Promise yourself that you will stop smoking just for three days . . . which is not really hard to do, and tell yourself that you are strong enough to do it.

3. Tell yourself that you will lose self-respect if you do not fulfil this promise, and encourage yourself by the thought that after three days of abstaining the backbone of the habit will be broken.

4. The next time you smoke, destroy your psychological pleasure by thinking negatively about smoking . . . (the main pleasure of smoking is psychological) . . . and you will find that you

*See page 133, Chapter 12.

have lost your craving. To think negatively, in this instance, means to dwell upon all the depressing consequences, the suffering and misery of lung cancer, of any lung damage, upon the humiliating position of being dependent on tobacco, even upon the expense of your bad habit.

5. To further strengthen your morale and determination, think positively about yourself and your character; how much better you feel being really master of yourself. Remember the old proverb ... "A master is not one who commands ten thousand slaves, it is he who is master of himself."

No one has ever really been cured of smoking by artificial means. The deterrent mixtures that are put in food or drink may produce sickness but some time later if a critical situation arises, the victim will probably start to smoke again. Only if he really wants to stop, if he stops by his own will-power can the cure be complete.

Fasting

In Chapter 5, *Purification*, we have written of partial fasting carried out in connection with seasonal rejuvenation and purification, but fasting is also observed at any time when the system needs a thorough cleaning.

Going without food is nature's way of resting and even repairing the body that has been over-taxed and over-worked. It is nothing to do with starving, which is to be *deprived* of necessary food. Fasting is undertaken voluntarily, either because the body cannot tolerate food ... as in serious illness where the whole mechanism is engaged in fighting for survival ... or because it is desired to get rid of accumulated impurities.

All animals, when they are ill, turn away from food. It is only civilized man who forces himself to eat when he would be better abstaining.

Some writers on yoga disapprove of the practice, claiming that if a proper diet is followed there should be no need for extra purification through fasting; but since we may assume that the majority do not follow a proper diet, an occasional one-day fast can do no harm, providing the person is not already very much underweight, and providing the fast can be done in suitable circumstances.

During a fast, rest as much as possible and go to bed early. Keep quiet, conserving all possible vital energy, not talking or even reading too much. You should take only water, or alternatively fruit juice, and an enema at the end of the day will help to get rid of impurities. The day after the fast you will feel fitter, younger and more energetic than ever.

5

PURIFICATION AND HYGIENE
CARE OF THE SKIN, EYES, EARS, HAIR, TEETH, SLEEP, REST AND RELAXATION

In the serious study of yoga, as followed in *ashrams*, the student cannot proceed to *pranayama* or breath control until his body has been purified. This is done by special diet, abdominal contractions, and by techniques which sometimes horrify Europeans. They include taking water into the bowels through the rectum, and swallowing lengths of cotton down into the stomach, withdrawing it after a certain time.

These last practices are not for the ordinary westerner, nor should they be attempted except under the guidance of an experienced teacher.

Although purification of the body is a necessary step on the yogi's path towards final liberation of the spirit, it is also a vital part of the method of delaying old age. We have already mentioned that modern geriatricians, as well as ancient yogis believe that incomplete elimination is a major cause of ageing.

Constipation and its consequent poisoning of the system may be rectified by diet and fasting, and through exercising the semi-voluntary muscles of the abdomen. These exercises, which may be learnt by anyone, provide deep internal massage.

The stomach contractions, *Uddiyana* and *Nauli* (pages124 and 151), should be practised every day, on an empty stomach, preferably first thing in the morning, before breakfast, even before drinking the fruit juice or cup of tea which many people take as soon as they wake up. They can easily be made a part of the ordinary morning routine, like cleaning the teeth or taking a shower. If time is short in the morning they may be done under the shower. (See also page 28.)

Other exercises which will give relief in the most stubborn cases of constipation are listed on page 28 but if the sufferer continues to stuff himself with unsuitable food, to grossly overeat and take no exercise he cannot expect complete success. An occasional fast, either water or fruit-juice, gives the body an excellent chance to rest and recover from the constant strain imposed on an overloaded digestion.

Traditionally, purification through fasts or partial fasts, is carried out at different seasons of the year, each one based on the same principle, but modified according to the natural foods available at that time.

The most important of these seasonal purifications is done in the spring. It is not only a spring-cleaning in the most literal sense, but a method of rejuvenation, for the student refreshes himself through rest and diet and also through uniting himself with nature in every way. He practises techniques for recharging himself through sun, ether, earth and water (page 86–7); he concentrates on the accumulation of vital energy; he goes to bed early and takes air-baths and sunbaths. He tries to confine himself to work as light as possible, while following the diet, and to waste none of his vitality in useless activities. He also practises many breathing exercises and spends much time in the open, consciously stepping into the rejuvenating cycle of spring.

It is usually the first week in spring that is dedicated to this purification.

On the first day a complete water fast should be observed; and an enema taken before going to bed.

On the second day *drink* only fruit juice; whatever you like, so long as you use only one kind of fruit.

On the third day, *eat* only fruit, either all citrus or all stone fruits, not mixing the two.

For the last four days of the week you may eat a diet of four ingredients . . . fruit, vegetables, nuts and honey. You may mix them if you like – there is no need to restrict yourself to one kind – but do not eat too much of anything. The maximum calorie intake should be 1,000 a day.

Care of the body

Outer and inner cleanliness are of equal importance. The skin itself is an organ. We breathe through the pores of the skin and if they become clogged the health suffers, sometimes seriously. There have been cases, some recently, of deaths caused by people painting themselves all over with gold paint and thus completely sealing the pores. This brings about poisoning of the system, as in failure of the kidneys.

Going to the other extreme, a too liberal opening of the pores can also be detrimental, especially to a sensitive skin. Too many Turkish baths and sauna baths do not suit everyone, particularly in dry climates or where people have the thin delicate skins bred in lands of soft mists and half-lights.

For the same reason, too much sun is bad for these fragile skins, which at best turn red and dry up into premature wrinkles, and at worst develop skin cancers.

Ordinary baths, or better still a shower, should be taken every day, and if this is not possible the whole body should be washed, not just face, neck and hands, as is sometimes done. Reluctance to undress is understandable in winter, but the belief that the inhabitants of cold countries need less washing than those in warmer climates is absurd and unfounded. In the tropics and sub-tropics people wear very few clothes and in many cases are frequently in the water . . . in rivers, lakes or the sea, the skin is ventilated and the perspiration runs unimpeded from the sweat glands; but in colder countries the body is constantly covered with thick clothes designed to keep the air from getting to the skin, which, unventilated, becomes clogged with discharges, while the clothes themselves, if not frequently changed, soon smell fusty and stale. A brief ride in a crowded Metro or Underground in winter demonstrates this point.

Sunbaths

Though excessive exposure is unwise, reasonable sunbathing is not only beneficial but essential for good health. The sun is our source of life; if our planet were a little closer or a little further from the sun there would be no life on it. It is the sun that ripens our fruit, vegetables and crops, that provides our vitamin D, that gives us warmth and vitality; but too much sun has the opposite effect, acting as a drug to the brain, sapping vitality and initiative.

If you live in a warm country or if you are able to spend your holidays in the sun, use some discretion. You cannot get a good tan in one day, you can only get sunburn, so it is pointless to roast yourself; nor should you expose yourself in the hottest part of the day. No one ever saw South Sea islanders or other tropical people sunbathing at that time. They prefer to rest in the shade and swim in the early morning or evening.

On the other hand, people who never expose their skins to

the sun at all are almost as foolish, unless of course it has been forbidden, as in cases of skin cancer.

Air baths

An air bath is taken like a sun bath, in a swimming costume, or if possible without any clothes at all, but lying in the shade. The object is to allow the whole skin of the body to breathe freely, as it cannot do when covered up with clothes.

Oil baths

The end of summer, or the spring are the best times for oil baths, though for dry and ageing skins they should be taken whenever possible. Warm the oil to body temperature . . . it may be any kind you like, the oilier the better . . . then take a warm shower to open the pores, and oil yourself from head to foot. Use as much oil as you can afford; if the skin is dry it will quickly soak in and disappear. The best way to complete the treatment is to wrap yourself in a large towel and take a sleep; or lie down and practice *Savasana* (page 107).

Regular exercise in the open air, apart from yoga *asanas*, should include walking, *in a relaxed way*, and swimming if possible.

Teeth

Middle-aged people often have strange ideas about their teeth. Sometimes their attitude is one of desperation and resignation; they seem to feel it expected of them to succumb to decay or gum conditions, to accept false teeth philosophically. Others have an almost insensate attachment to foul, decayed relics which they fight to save from extraction, permitting them to poison the whole system purely because they are their own.

It is better to have natural than false teeth but only if they are healthy and sound. If you still have your own teeth you should do everything possible to prolong their life through proper care.

They must be cleaned every day, preferably after each meal but at least before going to bed. Usually, cleaning is only done in the morning, and though it is an excellent custom and freshens the mouth for the day, it is less important than before bed, for it is during the night that much decay takes place.

Despite all the claims of advertisers, it is not tooth paste that stops decay but the mechanical action of removing food particles from between the teeth. (Primitive people sometimes clean their teeth with sand.) Brushing should be done carefully, using a downward stroke for the top teeth, and upward for the lower, in each instance moving the brush *away* from the gums. If the brushing is done towards them, or from side to side, recession of the gums will eventually result.

Rinsing out the mouth with salt and water is a substitute for brushing, if you should find yourself without a toothbrush, providing you swill the water vigorously round the teeth and gums. Massaging the gums with the finger – towards the tooth – will help prevent recession.

The teeth need blood, like every other part of the body; their nerves must be fed. All *asanas* that bring blood to the head will encourage healthy teeth and gums. (Headstand (page 123); Half-Candle (page 111); Head of a Cow (page 116); *Yoga-mudra* (page 115)). It is not advisable to bring extra blood to the head if a tooth is inflamed or abscessed. See also Chapter 11, page 129).

Cleaning the tongue

Before cleaning the teeth and before eating or drinking in the morning, clean your tongue of all the impurities that have collected on it during the night, which would otherwise be swallowed. Extend the tongue and scrape it carefully with the inverted bowl of a spoon. You will be surprised at the amount of deposit you can remove and your mouth will feel much fresher and cleaner.

Eyes

Too many middle-aged people take to glasses unnecessarily. One day, probably when tired or run down, they pick up the telephone book or newspaper and suddenly find they cannot focus. Since failing sight is so often taken as an inevitable part of life over forty they automatically assume that their time has come, and have themselves fitted out with glasses, upon which they soon become increasingly dependent.

An extraordinary number of otherwise intelligent men and

women overlook or are ignorant of the fact that the eyes are part of the body, like the stomach and lungs. It is generally accepted that if the whole system is in a lowered state, indigestion or perhaps heavy chest colds may develop; yet the eyes, ears and teeth are expected to carry on some autonomous life of their own and people become quite indignant when it is suggested that any disorder in these organs may be caused by poor general health.

The eyes are one of our main direct links with the outside world and carry constant stimulation and impressions to the brain. It is said that 50 per cent of our vitality is used when the eyes are open.

Assuming that there is no serious physical disease or defect, glasses could be avoided and good sight retained if the eyes are exercised regularly. The exercises given in Chapter 11 not only strengthen the eye muscles but improve the power of quick focusing.

Over thirty years ago Nancy Phelan was given glasses, on leaving school, to relieve "eye strain". Resenting her increasing dependence on them, she went to a pioneer teacher of eye-exercises and after 8 or 9 months found her eyes completely recovered. She has never had glasses since, though she uses her eyes constantly for reading, writing and photography, and her vision has never deteriorated. It was not until some years later that she discovered these exercises were identical with yoga eye exercises.

Good sight in old age is of the utmost importance. It is a disaster to be cut off, not only from reading, but from the faces one loves, the beauty of sea and sky and gardens at a time when one is becoming more in need of these things. Don't let this happen to you. Look after your eyes.

Never read in a bad light, especially if the print is small; in any case, such print should be avoided. Do not read with strong sunlight on the page, or with the light in your eyes. People used to say that cinemas (and now television) ruined the eyes, but providing they are not overdone, these entertainments need not be harmful. Do not stare at the screen. Exercise your eyes by moving them about, noticing details, following the action. From time to time change focus by moving them to a distant or closer point.

This changing of focus should also be done during any sustained close work. Raise your eyes from your drawing-board, typewriter or sewing machine and look out the window, or up at the ceiling . . . anywhere; it will relieve strain. Also practise palming whenever you can, even at your desk, shutting the eyes for a few seconds and putting the palms over them.

The habit of wearing dark glasses at all times is a kind of insanity. There are some people, mainly but not all women, who not only wear them in the house but also at night for dinner parties. As a fashion they are rather *démodé* and where the eyes are concerned they are ruinous. The only time sunglasses should be worn . . . and then they should be proper lenses . . . are in conditions of extreme brightness – the beach, the snow, a blinding white concrete road in summer. The more you wear them the more you will need them, until you will be as many people already are, like a mole, unable to tolerate sunlight at all.

If you live in a sunny climate you can strengthen your eyes and increase your tolerance of light by training. The Gilbertess, for instance, who live on tiny atolls of dazzling coral sand surrounded by brilliant, blinding tracts of ocean, do not need dark glasses, because for generations their eyes have been conditioned to this lighting.

Sunning the eyes

Sitting in Cross-legged or Diamond Pose (page 113) and with eyes closed, face the sun and move the head slowly from side to side, really letting it shine on your closed lids. After a few minutes quickly open and close them, but do not look directly at the sun.

Bathing the eyes

When the eyes are tired or inflamed, bathe them with warm water, or a very weak solution of boracic acid, or even cold weak tea, using an eye bath. It is particularly good for city people whose eyes are constantly exposed to dust, if it is not done too often. Women who use mascara on their lashes must be very careful to prevent it getting into the eyes and to remove it completely at night.

Blinking is nature's way of cleaning the eyes and is included in yoga eye exercises.

Staring, as a yoga exercise for strengthening the eyes is described on page 128 but staring in the ordinary sense is bad and strains the eyes. Blink and change focus from time to time.

Finally, *use your eyes*. Look at things. If you have ever lost your sight temporarily or feared this was going to happen you will know how extraordinarily fresh and beautiful everything seems, even the most mundane objects, when you look at them again. City people are usually too busy to look, unless it is organized looking in the form of an entertainment. They see, but it is a vision without dimension, without the quality of curiosity or wonder. Those who are growing older, who rush about less, who are no longer entirely preoccupied with getting and spending, need this habit of looking, of seeing things in the round.

We should not let ourselves become blind, like worms. The natural world is astonishingly beautiful and interesting. There are all kinds of little lives going on round us . . . birds, lizards, insects, the snail and caterpillar; things are growing, opening, developing and living; and even if we cannot get to the beach or the country or a city park, we can at least look up at the sky with its stars and moving clouds, using our eyes as though under the threat of losing them.

> "Look thy last on all things lovely,
> Every hour. Let no night
> Seal thy sense in deathly slumber
> Till to delight
> Thou have paid thy utmost blessing."

We should live by this poem all our lives, but never more so than when youth has gone.

The hair

Like teeth and waistlines, the hair is usually a vulnerable part of the middle-aged body; baldness has always been a traditional badge of ageing.

The scalp needs blood, but in most ageing bodies it gets less and less as the circulation slows down. This may be improved by the exercises and *asanas* on page 129.

The scalp also needs air to breathe. Men who wear hot felt hats in summer and women who spend the day doing house-work with their heads wrapped up in scarves, and go to bed with another scarf keeping the curling-pins in place are helping to destroy their hair.

If it is dry, do not wash it too often. For excessive dryness, rub in a little olive oil the night before washing. Do not let salt-water remain unrinsed. Massage the scalp as often as possible, with the tips of the fingers, and brush the hair regularly. (See Massage and Exercise on page 130.) Your hair reflects your general state of health, shining when you are well, becoming lank and dead when vitality is low.

There are many theories about greying hair, some people believing it is constitutional and hereditary, others that it comes from dryness, from washing in hot water, from vitamin deficiency. The inverted poses, particularly the Headstand, have been known to retard greying hair, and even, in some cases, have caused a fresh dark growth, replacing hair that had already turned white.

Ears

Certain *asanas* are recommended for keeping the ears healthy (page 129), through increasing the flow of arterial blood to the auditory nerves and generally toning up that area.

The ears should be kept clean and free of wax but if this is stubborn it should be removed by a doctor. On no account should you pour in or syringe strong solutions or hot oil, nor introduce into them any kind of instrument.

As with the eyes, *use* your ears. Listen. Try to hear not only the exhausting racket of the city round you but more subtle sounds – the wind in the trees, the sea, the birds. Listen to music. Though they may never become deaf in the literal sense, many people live their lives half-deaf, unable to hear anything but the most crude and obvious noises. If you cannot get to the country or the beach, go to a park where there is something to be heard other than traffic and loud voices. Best of all try, however difficult, to go occasionally to some place where you can be alone and listen to silence, for real silence is not just a negative absence of sounds; it is a living, positive entity; and in learning to listen to and love this living silence you may presently begin to hear something of your own essential self.

Several years ago a documentary film was made showing something of experiments with sleep as a rejuvenator. Old people in various stages of senility were put to sleep for long periods, and when finally woken, all displayed increased vigour and vitality, a more youthful appearance and a more alert attitude to life. If nothing else, these experiments confirmed what has so often been said; that sleep is the greatest restorer of all.

"Oh gentle sleep! Nature's soft nurse . . ." . . . "Oh sleep, it is a gentle thing beloved from pole to pole" . . . "Care-charming sleep . . ." . . . "Sleepe, that knitteth up the ravelled sleave of care . . ." "Meat for the hungry, drink for the thirsty, heat for the cold and cold for the hot . . ." the fact that so many poets wrote so feelingly about sleep indicates that creative artists are specially aware of their need of it. To some people it is more important than food. They live so intensely that by the end of the day their vitality is exhausted, and if sleep is withheld must fall back on their slender reserves. They have a chronic overdraft on their nervous energy, and prolonged deprivation of sleep usually brings bankruptcy in the form of a breakdown of some sort.

Even the most phlegmatic natures must have their share; and animals are no less dependent. Dogs kept awake for more than four nights will die.

But though sleep is nature's sweet nurse, it does not follow that great *quantities* are necessary, even for those who burn themselves up quickly, providing the *quality* is good enough. Many brilliant people doing highly responsible work can function on a few hours each night because they have mastered the art of sleeping properly. You may go to bed on your innerspring mattress in your city apartment after a tiring day in the office, sleep for eight or ten hours and wake up feeling jaded; yet after a day's gardening or walking in the country you can fall asleep for a few hours on a rather lumpy bed and next morning feel marvellously refreshed. In the country, despite your uncomfortable bed, the quality of your sleep was far higher than the ten hours you spent on your spring mattress. The healthy exercise in the open air, the peace and quiet round you while you slept all influenced your rest.

To improve the quality of sleep

If your sleep is bad, the surest way to make it worse is to worry about it. Remember that older people need less sleep than those who are growing or using up their vital energies in battling with life; and that there are many ways to overcome insomnia without recourse to sleeping pills.

Make sure that your room is as quiet as possible. Even in sleep we are influenced by sounds around us, which can, without waking us, destroy our rhythm. If you must sleep in a room near a busy street, put cotton-wool in your ears; and if you have the choice of two evils, choose a room where the noise is steady and continuous rather than erratic, for sudden loud bangs are worse than a sustained rumble.

If you cannot make your room really dark, sleep with a mask or a light scarf over the eyes; and do not sleep with high pillows, unless your health demands them.

Innerspring mattresses should be mounted on a wooden platform, not on another spring mattress, for too many springs can be as bad as none; and the bedclothes should be warm but light. Many people wake up exhausted after supporting a heavy load of covers all night. We use bedclothes in winter to prevent the dissipation of warmth given out by the body, so one well-insulated blanket or rug, though light in weight, is better than a pile of heavy objects that do not keep in the warmth.

Yoga teaches that the position of the bed can affect sleep. The magnetic current of the earth runs from north to south, and when the body, which is also a magnetic field, lies across it, e.g. from east to west, a disturbing effect is felt by nervous or sensitive people. If your sleep is uneasy it might be better to lie in the position recommended by yoga, in which the head is to the north and the feet to the south.

The state of mind has a great influence on ability to sleep and those who are a prey to anxiety, anger, resentment, jealousy, grief or worry of any kind usually suffer from insomnia. Overwork, over-excitement and staying up too late are other causes. No matter how interesting the book, how fascinating the television film, if you know you have reached the critical moment when you could fall asleep, you must go to bed. Dozing in the chair is no good at all, for when you do get to bed you will find you are wide awake again and will probably lie all night tossing and turning, or fall into an exhausted early-morning stupor that leaves you feeling worse than before.

It is not reasonable to expect to sleep immediately if your mind is stimulated by work or entertainment. If you are a bad sleeper, try to slow down a little before bedtime. Listen to music, relax, take a warm bath, or best of all, do some deep breathing by the open window.

Hunger can keep you awake, just as much as over-eating; indigestion is a common cause of insomnia. People eat heavy meals at night, when their bodies are too tired to digest them, then lie awake for hours wondering why they cannot sleep. If the meal has been accompanied or followed by a family row or argument there is even less chance of sleep, for the nerves will be tensed, the mind agitated and the stomach feel as though tightened into a hard knot.

Try to eat less at night, unless you are in the habit of staying up long enough to digest it; and cut out rich and heavy foods which would tax anyone's digestion at any hour of the day.

If you are given to falling asleep early, then waking at about three or four in the morning and being unable to sleep again, do not lie fretting about it. Either profit from the rest . . . relaxing your muscles, practising deep breathing or *Savasana*, or trying to think *agreeable* thoughts; or put on the light and read a book. Very likely you will go to sleep over it; and if not, it will not really matter. You have had the best part of the night, for the most refreshing sleep comes before midnight. Remember again that you do not need so much sleep as you get older; and that people do not go mad or have nervous breakdowns for the loss of a few hours. What is far more harmful is worrying about your insomnia.

There are certain *asanas* and exercises which have a direct influence upon the ability to sleep. These are *Savasana* (page 107); Spinal Massage (page 95) and Triangular Pose, or Pose of Tranquillity (page 111). Some students say that the Shoulderstand and Headstand before bed have helped them; but deep breathing done by an open window will soothe anyone's nerves, and *Savasana*, practised when you are in bed, will continue the process. Try also deep breathing in bed with the finger-tips on the solar plexus. The rhythmical rise and fall of the stomach has a soothing and hypnotic effect.

The quality of the sleep may also be improved by constant proper respiration. Yoga ensures this, even in sleep. Though no one stays in the same position all night, whatever pose they adopt is either on the right side, left side, back or stomach. If we train ourselves to breathe properly in these positions while awake, the body will automatically turn on this complete breathing when we lie in them while asleep.

The positions are:

1. Lying flat on the back.
2. On the right side with the right knee bent, right arm extended under the head and left arm lying loosely behind the back.
3. The same as (2), lying on the left side.
4. Lying flat on the stomach with head turned to one side and arms limply by the sides.

Rest and relaxation

An annual holiday is a good idea but it is not the solution for everyone, particularly people who use up their vital energy quickly, who drive themselves and live intensely.

A short holiday, even a few days, several times a year is better for them than staggering along under a twelve months' accumulation of exhaustion, and finding themselves too tired or overwrought to enjoy the break when it comes. It is very common to hear people say their two or three weeks' holiday was not enough, that they were barely starting when they had to go back to work.

One of our insanities is that a working man takes his holiday not when he needs it most but when it is his turn or it suits the boss or there is a slack period at work, or some other artificial reason. The fact that he is so tired that his work suffers does not seem to matter.

Eventually employers will learn that everyone is not the same and what suits a phlegmatic man is not good for a sensitive or highly-strung temperament, and something will be done to improve the situation; but in the meantime those who cannot take a needed holiday will find help in learning to relax through *Savasana*, through breathing cycles, through improving the quality of their sleep and regular recharging of vital energy.

We in the West have been brought up with the idea that to be inactive is to waste time and that this is shocking and wrong. It is time to discard this nonsense. Everyone should learn to waste a little time, not to be always busy or rushing or organized; to do nothing and enjoy it without a sense of guilt. *"What is this life, if full of care, We have no time to stand and stare?"*

6

SEX IN MIDDLE AGE

When it is said that the practice of *Hatha* yoga prolongs the creative part of life, the powers of physical procreation are included as well as those of intellect, imagination and initiative.

Although most yogis of the East observe strict celibacy to conserve and increase all physical and nervous energy, there are certain schools believing that liberation of the spirit comes through release of the sexual impulse,* and various techniques are designed and practised for this purpose.

Sometimes in middle-age there is a failing of virility and a loss of sexual drive. Such disabilities may be avoided, or improved if they occur, and sex enjoyed even at an advanced age – by western standards – if the sex glands are kept healthy and active, the body in good condition and the supply of vital energy not allowed to diminish. Yoga practice ensures all these; and proper diet, adequate rest and the cultivation of a relaxed attitude help to maintain the good health, confidence and attractive appearance that contribute to a satisfactory sex life.

The nervous tension or exhaustion so destructive to harmonious relationships can be overcome by *Savasana* (page 107) and by breathing cycles. Sexual energy and drive are strengthened by the Headstand (page 123), Shoulderstand (page 110), Half-shoulderstand (page 111), Head-to-knee Pose (page 120), Eagle (page 117), Plough (page 119), Fish (page 121), Spinal Twist (page 120), *Aswini mudra* (page 116), *Uddiyana* (page 124). Vital energy is increased by Energy-charging breathing cycles; *vajroli mudra* (page 116), Circulating Life Force (page 84) and Transmuting of Energies (page 72). The Raised Poses in the Appendix will contribute to greater confidence, and full general practice will keep the whole body in the best possible condition.

*Sexual intercourse practised for liberation in Tantric schools is in the nature of a rite, and is preceded by intense physical and spiritual preparation and purification. The yogi must be in the highest state of physical development, with his body under complete control of his mind. It is said that he must have mastery over the *bindu* (semen), meaning ability to prolong coitus without permitting ejaculation. Coitus liberates, but the loss of sperm is detrimental to mental powers. If the *bindu* does "fall" he has techniques for drawing it back again into his body.

Such mental exercises as Sorting Seeds of Thought, I am Master of Myself, I am Stronger than Fear, help develop a more positive and optimistic attitude, which will complement improved physical well-being.

Change of life, male and female
Menopause in women

Change of life in women is known as the menopause, the time when the process of menstruation ceases, either suddenly or gradually, bringing the end of the child-bearing period. It is sometimes accompanied by disturbing and distressing symptoms, physical and psychological, ranging from hot flushes, giddiness, palpitations and loss of energy, to depression, failing memory, insomnia, increased nervous tension and irritability, which in extreme cases can cause complete loss of mental balance.

Women who have led busy active lives seem to suffer less than those who have always been spoilt and indolent and whose sole attention has always been focused on themselves and their ailments. Some women really do make the most of their change of life, using it as a kind of blackmail, an excuse for every little self-indulgence and selfishness and sometimes dragging it out far longer than justified. Although a definite physical change does occur – one set of glands going out of action and others taking over in compensation – and the balance of the body is upset in the process, the menopause is no more an illness than pregnancy, and it is better not to brood about it, though when there is actual physical suffering proper care should be taken.

Middle-aged women all over the world are now helping themselves to weather this period of their lives through yoga. On the physical side, apart from improving the general state of health, they find much relief in practising *Savasana*; in breathing cycles for relaxing nervous tension; the Triangular Pose and rocking exercise (page 95) for insomnia; the Shoulderstand, for hot flushes; *Uddiyana*, Head-to-knee and the digestive cycle for indigestion and constipation, and *Pavanamuktasana*, or knee-to-stomach position for flatulence (page 123). *Uddiyana*, and if possible, *Nauli*, Cobra and Locust will also help in menstrual difficulties, though during the actual period it is better to suspend practice and concentrate on rest.

A diet in which over-stimulating food and drink are reduced

– preferably discarded – proper elimination, plenty of rest and fresh air are also important.

There are various ways of improving psychological troubles, one of the best being to keep the mind fully occupied and absorbed in interests outside oneself – work, hobbies, people; and there are mental exercises which if practised seriously will bring increased calmness, balance and greater serenity. Change of life should be regarded constructively, not dwelling upon the loss of physical charms, the encroachment of old age that some women regard as inevitable, and which breed lack of confidence, depression, self-pity and a sense of rejection; but realizing that such gloomy thoughts are only a symptom of the general condition, which will pass, and which can be controlled; that the menopause does not mean loss of feminine attraction or the end of a woman's romantic life; and that usually, after it is over, there is an extraordinary upsurge of new energy – as though, having finished with the ordeal, the body feels it can start again and take a fresh interest in life.

Change of life in men

Change of life also occurs in men, although it is a more individual process than in women; and as with women, a well-adjusted man whose life is full of interest is less likely to suffer than one who has always been negative, ineffectual and sorry for himself.

Sometimes the change begins in the mind. Having over-worked and neglected his body for years, the man notices a diminution of energy, a loss of youthful drive and its attendant optimism. He becomes depressed and starts to view himself and his life pessimistically. Even men who have attained material success may be affected this way, seeing their achievements as worthless or insignificant, while those who have accomplished less see themselves as failures. Unhappily, men more than women are affected by the primitive conventions of our society, which regards a man as a failure if he has not made money, no matter how successful his personal life.

Whatever the cause, the victim feels he has failed. He broods, becomes gloomy, irritable, unreasonable, defeated. His mental state affects his body. He is always tired; he has chronic indigestion; he cannot sleep; he becomes impotent. He feels his life is over.

In other men the process is reversed. Due to physical exhaustion, worry or inadequate diet (with possible vitamin deficiency), they find that their virility is declining. Though this may be only a temporary state it is often taken as permanent. Instead of trying to correct it the sufferer worries, and the more he worries the worse the condition becomes. He may take to alcohol as escape; he may just become unbearable and unfit to live with; he sometimes even allows it to poison his life and ruin his marriage.

Other men again are affected differently. They become restless; they are suddenly assailed by a sense of time rushing past, of opportunities missed, of approaching extinction. To prove how young they are, they turn to younger and younger women, sometimes with tragic consequences.

It has been said that when sex fails many men feel their life is over. This is only half-true; it is when it fails *prematurely* that a man becomes distressed, and this need never happen if he has kept himself in good condition. Even when temporary impotence does occur it can be improved and finally overcome if the sufferer has the patience and determination to help himself.

Physical improvement through yoga is brought about by practising the Headstand, for its effect on the pituitary, and the Shoulderstand, for its effect on the thyroid, since both these glands have a great influence on the sex glands. *Vajroli mudra* and *Aswini mudra* are also important; the energy-charging techniques on pages 82–7 and the increasing of sexual energy through transmutation described on page 72.

Savasana and breathing cycles help relieve the tension that may be contributing to the trouble, and mental exercises leading to increased confidence, inner strength, and a positive attitude should also be practised, since in impotence a negative state of mind can be physically inhibiting. Sometimes a little common sense is also required, as in women's change of life, for male pride can be an impediment to overcoming the complaint. Men have prolonged their disability unnecessarily through a belief that their wives are condemning, even despising them, ignoring the fact that no mature or intelligent woman would sit in judgement on a man for a temporary failure of this kind, any more than she would expect him to blame her for some physical weakness of her own.

Sublimation of energies

Very little is known in the West about yoga teaching concerning the energies in the body.

The five energies are – Mental, Physical and Sexual Energies, Energy of the Intellect, and Energy of the Soul. Of these, the first three are interchangeable or transmutable; the fourth is independent; and the fifth is also independent and indestructible.

Yoga teaches that the fourth Energy (Intellect or Personality), which is the quality that makes each one of us different from the others, is already fully grown at birth and cannot be developed further. Energy of the Soul is the divine spark, the touch of God in man.

Since the first three Energies are transmutable, physical energy may be transformed into mental or sexual energy; and sexual into physical or mental energy.

Many methods of effecting these transmutations are regularly practised in *ashrams* and monasteries in the East. Some advanced forms of yoga, such as *Kundalini* yoga (see page 77) demand such intense accumulation of mental powers that every other possible form of energy must be drawn from the body to strengthen the mind. Sexual energy is transmuted into mental energy for this purpose, which is why a highly advanced yogi must be completely celibate.

Although ordinary men and women are not concerned with such practices, many could find relief through simplified methods of sublimation. The transmuting of sexual energy into purely physical energy is recommended when no natural outlet is available, for repression of sex is bad. It can lead to warped personalities, bitterness and unhappiness, and to many mental and physical disorders, but transmutation to another form of energy is beneficial, for it not only relieves pressure but increases physical or mental powers, personal magnetism and dynamic force. Through sublimation, sexual energy that can find no natural expression is used harmlessly and constructively.

Determination, perseverance and faith in the power of the method are the main requirements for success. It is also very important that existing physical energy should be at a high level, and as a preliminary, a number of breathing exercises for recharging the solar plexus should be practised. (Chapter 9 – Breathing) (see page 115 (Dangerous Pose).)

Transmuting of Sex energy to Physical energy

Sit down, in the cross-legged position, establish rhythmical breathing as instructed in Chapter 12, *Mental Techniques,* and concentrate on the thought of sublimation. Form a mental image of the sex energy being drawn up from its customary seat,* with each inhalation, and directed, with each exhalation, to the solar plexus, where it is stored as increased physical energy.

The exercise is also practised in the Shoulderstand or Headstand positions, in which the Region of the Moon is raised above the Region of the Sun. This speeds up the recharging process.

Transmuting Sex energy to Mental energy

Sex Energy may be transmuted into Mental Energy by the same means.

After the pose and breath are established, imagine that with each incoming breath you are drawing sex energy from the Moon Region and directing it, with each outgoing breath, up *through the spine* to the head, where it manifests as increased power of the mind.

This is also done in crossed-legged pose or in Shoulderstand or Headstand, using the same principle.

Transmuting Physical energy to Sex energy

For those whose life permits normal sex activity but who perhaps feel their powers in this direction are failing, physical energy may be transmuted into increased sex activity. The same procedure is used, in reverse. With inhalation the energy is drawn *from* the solar plexus, and directed, with exhalation, *to* the region of the sex organs, with recharging effects.

*The seat of sexual energy is the region of the sex organs, in yoga called the Moon Region. The seat of physical energy is the solar plexus, the Region of the Sun.

7

THE DIFFERENT PATHS OF Y

In youth and early middle-age most householders are absorbed in earning a living, breeding, providing for the family, managing their affairs, but when the demands of these activities subside they often feel a need for something more, something they cannot define.

This could be the best age at which to study yoga, for behind its physical aspects is an ancient philosophy which has brought meaning into many lives.

Yoga means union – union of man's individual spirit with the spirit of the universe or God, but there is more than one method of achieving this union. All methods lead to the same goal; they are different ways to travel; for due to *karmic** laws and individual stages of development all men were not suited for the same path. Though each of these yogic paths is distinguished by its particular practices they cannot be rigidly classified or put into watertight compartments. They overlap, merge and become diffused at certain points of training.

Hatha yoga is the path of bodily strength and control; *Karma* yoga, the path of right action; *Bahkti* yoga, the path of devotion; *Gnani* yoga, the path of knowledge; *Rajah* yoga brings complete mastery of the mind, and *Kundalini* yoga the development of higher faculties.

Spiritual enlightenment is not dependent on intellect or education; too much of either can sometimes be an impediment, inhibiting the surrender necessary for true illumination. Liberation of the spirit comes only through suspension of the mind; therefore, though scholars and men of great mental gifts and attainments are drawn to yoga, lack of formal education or a sense of intellectual inadequacy are no disqualification. There is something above intellect, something which we can only call intuition in its highest sense, a direct channel to divinity. This, with sincerity, an open mind, a capacity for belief and a desire to

Karmic law.
The law of cause and effect. It is directly connected with the laws of reincarnation, and teaches that our present life can be influenced by actions – right and wrong – done in previous lives. It also provides for the exercise of Free Will, by which a man may, through noble living and right action, overcome karmic influence.

ow, are the essentials without which no one can succeed.

Yoga is so ancient that we have no definite knowledge of its origins. It is recorded in the Vedas, the oldest books in the world, written 2,500 years before Christ, but much earlier figures of yogis in meditative poses have been found, suggesting that its real age is even greater.

The traditional belief is that true knowledge is only given to those who are capable of receiving it; to sages who have attained the highest stage of spiritual advancement. These are the great *mahatmas*, or spiritual guides, and it is through them that the teachings are handed down to their chosen pupils, who spend years studying with their teacher (*guru*). Many of these *chelas* or pupils have travelled hundreds of miles to find their teacher; some are brought to them in strange ways; but it is for the *guru* to decide whether or not he will accept the pupil, and his decision is made on purely spiritual grounds.

No one seeking to study yoga for commercial exploitation or material gain is accepted; and though in India, as in the West, there are false yogis, the true masters still exist. They are not found exhibiting themselves on the roadside or in the bazaars; they are hidden away from the world, so hard to find that many sincere seekers have failed to trace them. But yoga comes to those who really desire it. It is said that "when the pupil is ready the teacher appears".

Hatha Yoga

Liberation through *Hatha* Yoga involves bringing the body to its highest state of development and under complete control of the mind. It could be a starting point for all other yogas, in the sense that a healthy body is an asset when undergoing any form of training, just as a musical instrument gives a better performance when it is properly tuned.

The word *Hatha* comes from two Sanskrit roots . . . *ha*, which means the sun, and *tha*, meaning the moon. It is said that the sun controls the breath flowing through the right nostril, while the flow through the left nostril is controlled by the moon. *Yoga*, used in this context, means the union of the two breaths . . . the basis of the whole system.

Traditionally, there are eight steps to follow: abstinences; observances; *asanas* or bodily poses; breath control; withdrawal of mind from external influences; concentration; contemplation and identification.

74

The abstinences and observances (*yamas* and *niyamas*) must be strictly kept by students of ascetic yoga schools; but they need not be so rigidly enforced in the case of ordinary householders who practise *Hatha* yoga for physical well-being.

The abstinences (*yamas*) are: Refraining from violence or causing pain in any way by word or deed to others or to oneself.

Refraining from lying, directly or indirectly, by word or action.

Refraining from stealing, which includes the taking of bribes.

Chastity.

Non-possession (refraining from possessiveness in any sense).

The observances or *niyamas* are:

Purity, in body, thought and action.

Contentment; a philosophical acceptance of whatever life brings.

Austerity; physical austerity . . . the ability to bear hardship and pain, the development of inner strength and mental control; and self-development – which includes study and meditation.

The fifth observance is devotion to God.

The practice of these *yamas* and *niyamas* is also known as *kriya yoga*.

The *asanas* or bodily poses of *Hatha* yoga – 84 in number – include those given in this book; and we have also touched upon breath control or *pranayama*. Advanced *pranayama* techniques should only be imparted by a teacher, for they are dangerous to mental balance and to life itself if practised without proper guidance and preliminary purification.

Withdrawal means the detachment of the mind from external stimuli, the switching off of the perceptionary powers. It leads to control of the senses and mental and spiritual advancement.

Concentration is when the attention is kept focused upon one point. It brings power to still the mind, and leads to *Contemplation*, in which the thoughts are turned upon every aspect of the contemplated object. *Identification* is a state of such extreme concentration that the personality becomes merged with the object of contemplation. Identification with all and everything is liberation of the spirit: – *samadhi*.

Karma Yoga

Karma yoga is a very practical path for men and women who must lead an active life as householders in a materialistic society. It does not require withdrawal from the world, nor impose any rigid training or austerities. It is the yoga of work and right action.

The *karma* yogi works as hard as he can, but freely, not enslaved by the desire to acquire more possessions or defeat a rival or obtain greater power. He enjoys the material fruits of his work, providing he has obtained them honourably and without injury to others, but at heart he remains unattached and free, however much pleasure his possessions bring him.

This is not a philosophy only suitable for the East. During the last war hundreds of ordinary Londoners learnt a form of non-attachment, discovering that material possessions were comparatively unimportant when the issue was life or death. Each morning, after the air raid, people who had lost everything felt themselves fortunate because they had their lives; and the extraordinary spirit that prevailed at that time in the bombed city was the expression of a strange, albeit unconscious, sense of freedom from material bondage.

Gnani Yoga

This is the yoga that attracts intellectuals and philosophers, those who must know the reason behind everything, the secrets of creation. It is a difficult and lonely path, for its demands are too great for the average man.

The *gnani* yogi steps aside from life as we live it and dedicates himself to finding truth through the highest form of thought, endlessly questioning all accepted concepts. He is withdrawn and detached, not only from society but from his own personality; in a sense, like a man who chooses to live in an iron lung, using it but not regarding it as part of himself nor holding himself responsible for it.

In terms of western life the *gnani* yogi might be compared to a dedicated scholar, untidy and absorbed; or an absent-minded professor who is never quite aware of his surroundings.

Bahkti Yoga

The yoga of love and devotion, which appeals to those who live more by emotion than intellect. It is often suggested that since devotion is implicit in all other yogas, *Bahkti* is not a separate path, though its followers regard it as such.

This is the most popular yoga among the people of India, for it makes no great intellectual demands and requires no special training. It appeals to man's instinctive need to love, and recognizes love of all kinds as a form of worship – whether between lovers, parents and children, or friends; whether a wide love of all humanity or for God himself. It is the force of love evoked that is important, and that is regarded as a divine manifestation.

It is the path for the simple and devout soul; the yoga of the heart.

Kundalini Yoga

The study and practice of rousing the latent higher faculties of the mind, which otherwise would only be developed after thousands of years of evolution.

Kundalini, or latent nervous energy, is described as a "coiled serpent sleeping at the base of the spine", and when she is woken, by the appropriate practices, "she uncoils, and rushes, hissing, up through the spine to the top of the brain".

On her journey from her sleeping-place, she passes through the six *chakras** of the body, arousing each one in turn. With each *chakra* "in vibration" the yogi experiences the awakening of different psychic powers.

Much has been written about *Kundalini* and attempts have been made to explain the phenomenon in purely physical terms. It has been suggested that she is the right vagus nerve of the sympathetic nervous system and that the psychic powers are awakened by connecting the *chakras* with the conscious mind. Whatever the explanation, these powers exist. They are occasionally encountered in people who appear to have been born with them, e.g. mediums, clairvoyants, diviners, and those with fantastic talent for instant calculation.

Rajah Yoga

Royal yoga, the highest or Prince of yogas, is often described as the last stage of development, and like *gnani*, is for the few rather than the majority.

Rajah yoga is concerned with the attainment of full power and control of the mind. It embraces the accumulation of knowledge

Chakras: Nervous plexuses, psychic centres. See Chapter 12, page 143.

(*gnani* yoga), the unfolding of psychic powers (*Kundalini* yoga), esoteric experience, meditation and philosophy. It is the yoga of wisdom, balance, control and mergence.

In our own times Einstein and Bertrand Russell might be described as *rajah yogis* in the sense that their mental development is far superior to that of the ordinary man.

There are other yogas . . . the yoga of sounds, of geometrical forms, of controlling natural forces, of penetrating other dimensions . . . but whatever path he follows, the true yogi is always striving for one objective – the state in which the barriers of mind and body fall away and permit him, while still in this flesh, to liberate his spirit.

The Siddhis or Attainments

The *siddhis* or attainments of the yogi are suprahuman powers over the laws of nature. They are brought about by the harnessing of all powers, within and without, through intense concentration. The principle behind them is that since man and the universe are manifestations of the same force, he can learn to control this force, whether in his own body or in the world around him.

Samadhi

Samadhi is the superconscious state in which conscious and subconscious minds are submerged and in which the individual soul is united with the soul of the universe.

The yogi who has attained superconsciousness can descend from it to the conscious state again, but he knows how to re-enter *samadhi* at will. When his cycle on earth is finished he enters into *maha-samadhi* from which he does not return. *Maha-samadhi*, which we in the West regard as physical death, is brought about by stopping the heart, through control of the breath.

No one has ever described *samadhi*, since words are an expression of the mind and in this state the mind plays no part . . . it is left behind by the spirit as the launching tower is left when the rocket takes off. Yet we can dimly guess at it. The sense of belonging in the fullest sense, of being at one with the whole universe; complete assurance that all is well; the feeling that the natural world, the stars, sea, mists, the trees, are all part of oneself as one is part of them; complete absorption . . . union

. . . identification, and an absolute *knowing*, in which reason, thought, logic play no part . . . all these, intensified and magnified to the highest degree, and with them the peace of God that passeth understanding . . . It has sometimes been described as Bliss. Certainly those who know it are changed for ever, serene and assured.

8

BREATHING

The most important message of physical yoga . . . that to control breath is to control life force, and perhaps life itself . . . could completely revolutionize our way of life.

In the *ashrams*, *shalas* (yoga schools) and monasteries of the East, where the art of breathing has been practised and taught for centuries, strange stories are told of what has been achieved through breath control, by sages of the past. Apart from its remarkable healing and invigorating powers, it is the key to the mysterious power of levitation (ability to defy gravity forces), and, it is said, is the means whereby the ancient wise men could travel through the air with the speed of an arrow.

Nicholas Roerich, the Russian artist, philosopher and mystic, who lived in Tibet for many years, claimed to have seen monks travelling through space; and at an island *ashram* in the South China Sea, Michael Volin was shown a flat stone protruding from the top of a sheer cliff, and told that from this platform sages used to take off into the air for their morning promenade.

These stories are told, not to suggest that readers could learn to float in the air, but to emphasize the tremendous potentialities of breath control.

Four attainments of controlled breath could be learnt by any serious student.
They are:

1. Recharging the body when physical energy is at a low ebb.
2. Ability to pacify the mind and entire nervous system by breathing.
3. Warming up the body when cold.
4. Cooling the body when hot.

In healing yoga, controlled breath is used for self-healing and to benefit others. By tradition, this method is always taught by personal instruction and can only be briefly described here (page 91).

The majority of the breathing techniques are devoted to the accumulation of vital energy, for it is this vital energy, or *prana* that holds the body together. When it diminishes the ageing process quickly sets in. People become less active, consciously

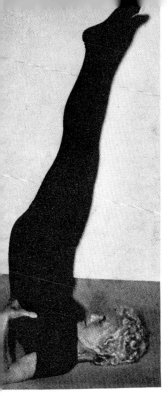

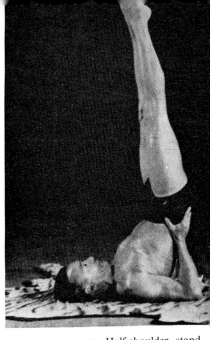

PLATE 2 : Half-shoulder stand or Half Candle

PLATE 1 : Shoulder stand or Candle

PLATE 3 : Pose of Tranquillity (Triangular Pose)

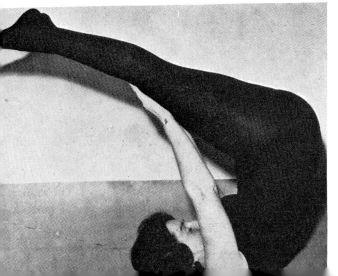

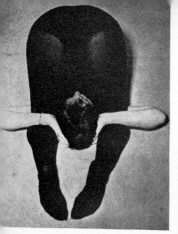

PLATE 4 : Choking Pose

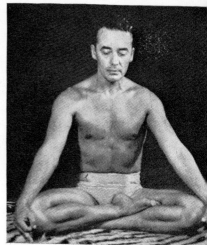

PLATE 5 : Pose of an Adept

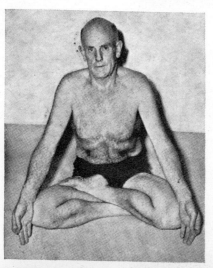

PLATE 6 : Half-lotus

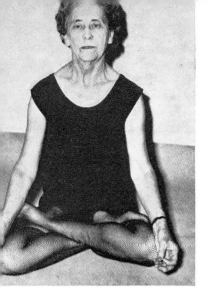

PLATE 7 : Lotus position

PLATE 8 : Diamond Pose

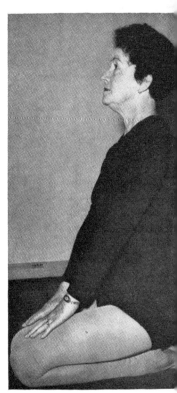

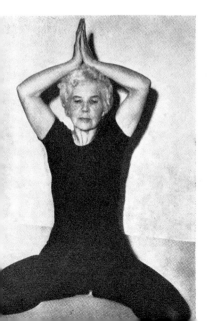

PLATE 9 : Pose of a Frog

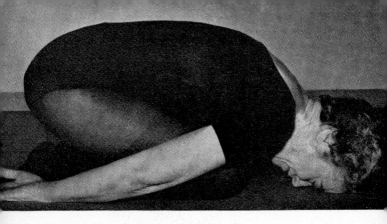

PLATE 10 : Pose of a Child

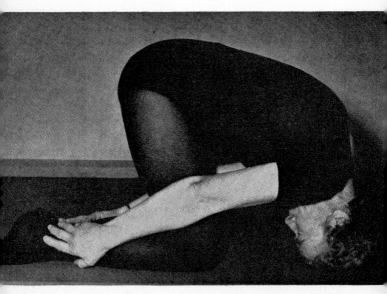

PLATE 11 : Pose of a Hare

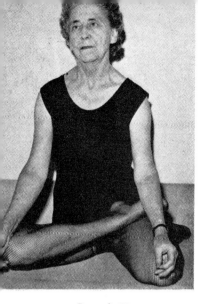

PLATE 12 : Pose of a Hero

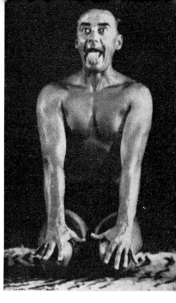

PLATE 13 : Pose of a Lion

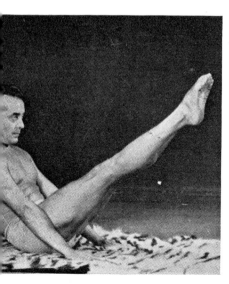

PLATE 14 : *Vajroli mudra*

PLATE 15 : Head of a Cow Pose

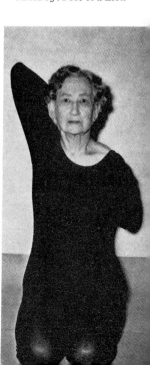

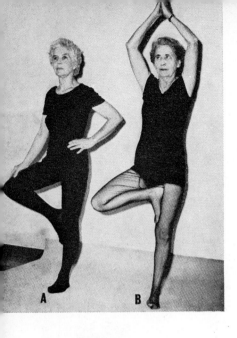

PLATE 16: Balancing

A   B

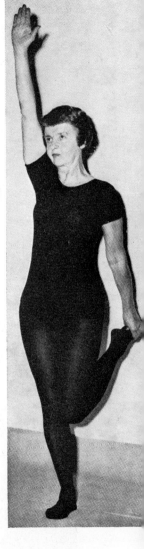

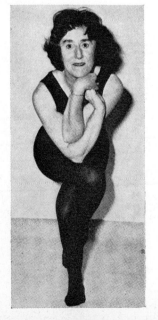

PLATE 17: Pose of a Tree

PLATE 18: Pose of an Eagle

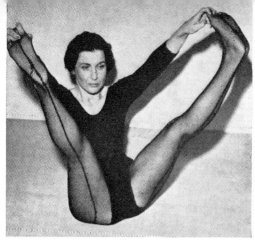

PLATE 19 : Angular Pose

PLATE 20 : Arch Gesture

PLATE 21 : Stretching –
cross-legged

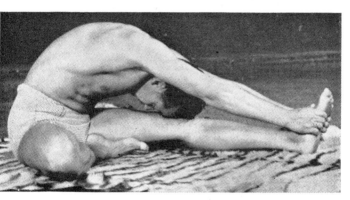

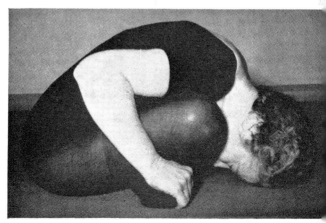

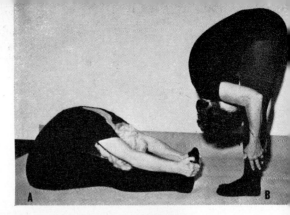

PLATE 22:
Head to Knee

PLATE 23:
Star Pose

PLATE 24:
Plough Pose

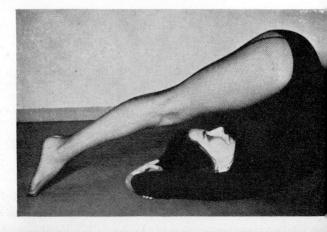

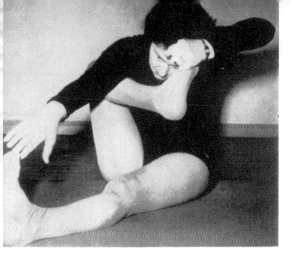

PLATE 25 :
Archer

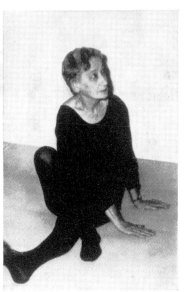

PLATE 26 : Little Twist

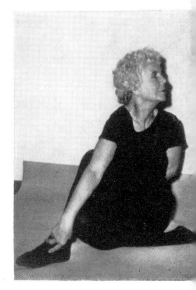

PLATE 27 : Spinal Twist

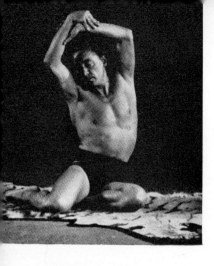

PLATE 28 : Sideways Swing

PLATE 29 :
Modification of Fish Pose

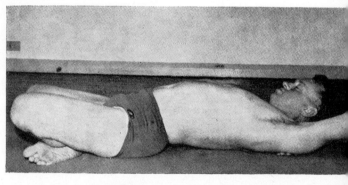

PLATE 30 :
Cobra

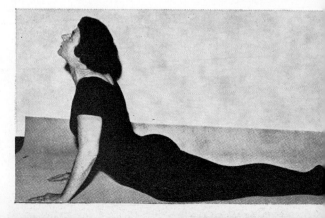

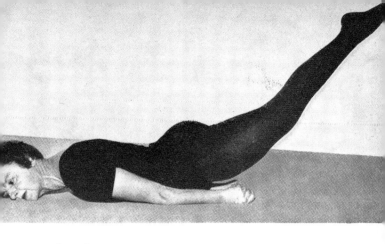

PLATE 31 : Locust

PLATE 32 : Pose of a Camel

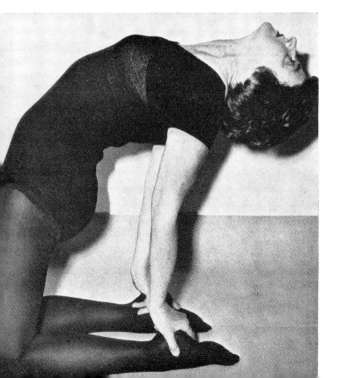

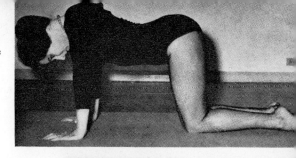

PLATE 33 : Pose of a Cat

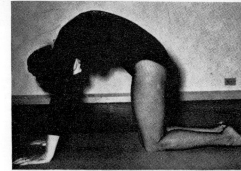

PLATE 34 : Pose of a Cat

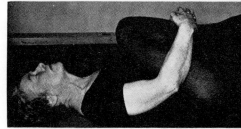

PLATE 35 : Knees to stomach

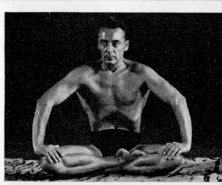

PLATE 36 : *Uddiyana*

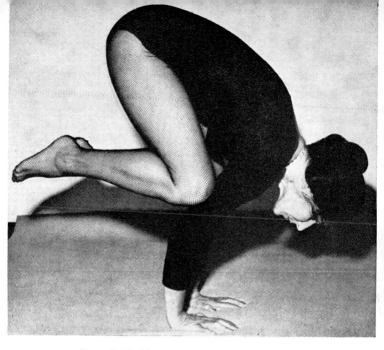

PLATE 37 : Pose of a Bird (*age* 51)

PLATE 38 : Pose of a Raven (*age over* 50)

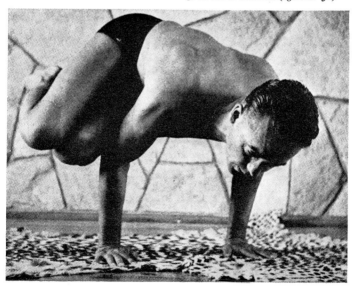

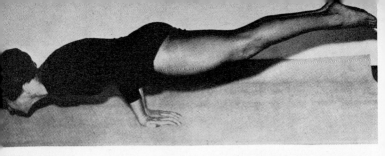

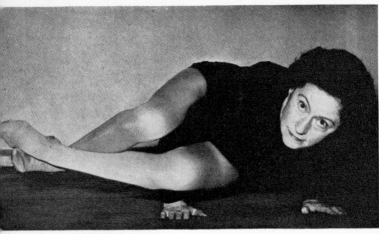

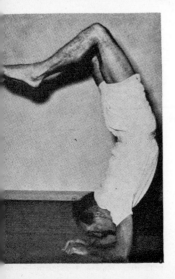

PLATE 39 : Peacock (*age* 51)

PLATE 40 : Pose of Eight Curves (*age* 60)

PLATE 41 : Scorpion (*age* 58)

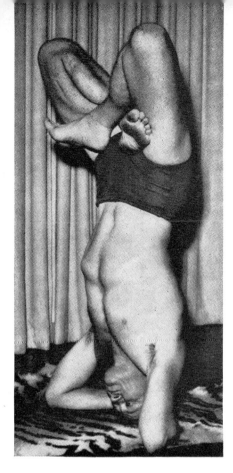

PLATE 42 :
Bound Headstand (*age* 48)

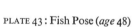

PLATE 43 : Fish Pose (*age* 48)

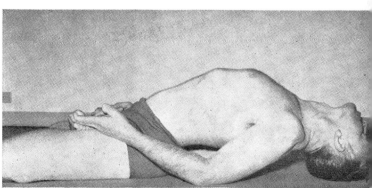

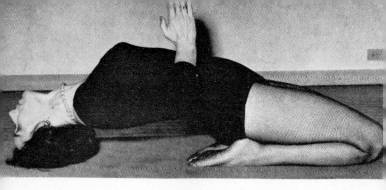

PLATE 44:
Supine Pelvic (*age* 51)

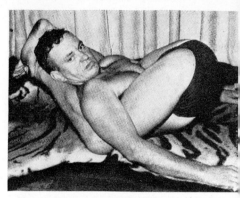

PLATE 45 : Noose Pose (*age* 48)

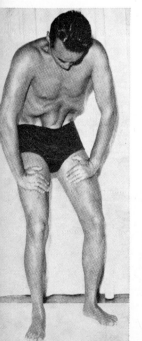

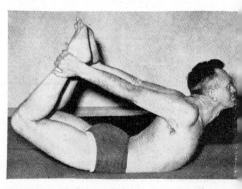

PLATE 46 : Bow Pose (*age* 48)

PLATE 47 : *Nauli* (*age over* 50)

and unconsciously trying to spare their bodies. This leads to atrophy of muscles, flabbiness, wrong posture, protruding stomachs, prolapses, and other complaints associated with old age. In some countries geriatricians now advocate regular breathing exercise as as a means of prolonging life.

We have already explained (page 21) that by increasing the volume of *inhalation*, the intake of *prana* is increased; and that with *exhalation* it could be directed by will-power and concentration to the solar plexus (the seat of vital energy) or to any other part of the body. The extra amount of *prana* inhaled makes all the difference to physical well-being.

Prana is also accumulated in the solar plexus while breath is *retained*, the student learning to separate life force from the air by concentration.

Through deep breathing, the oxygenation of the bloodstream is improved, and every vital organ, endocrinal gland, nervous centre and body tissue receives better nourishment. To breathe correctly is to stay young longer.

How to breathe correctly

In yoga breathing the lungs are completely filled and completely emptied. This is quite unlike usual shallow breathing in which only the top part of the lungs is used.

With *inhalation*, let your stomach come out, inflating it like a frog. This lowers the diaphragm and fills the bottom of the lungs. Expand the lower part of the chest, filling the lungs further. Raise the middle part of chest, slightly contracting the stomach, and finally lift and expand the upper ribs, filling the top part of the lungs.

In *exhalation* the process is reversed. The stomach is drawn in, the diaphragm is lifted and the expanded ribs relax, resulting in complete emptying of the lungs.

Although we have described the process in stages it is done as one smooth continuous movement.

The best way to accustom yourself to this method, which most people find the exact reverse of their ordinary breathing, is to put your hands on your abdomen, with finger-tips touching, and practice rhythmical inhaling and exhaling through the nose. If you are doing it properly the finger-tips should move apart as you inhale and come together again with exhalation.

The tempo of yoga breathing is much slower than the normal

rate . . . five–six breaths to the minute instead of fifteen to twenty. Practise counting six as you inhale, six as you exhale. Slowing the breath slows down and rests the heart, pacifies the nerves and relaxes the whole system.*

A very simple exercise in learning rhythmical breathing is to sit with the finger on the pulse, counting six pulse-beats for inhalation; retain the breath for three heart-beats; exhale counting six, and retain emptiness for three.

When this complete yoga breath is mastered, and an ability to concentrate is developed, the actual breathing exercises may be practised.

Recharging Breaths

Recharging cycles usually comprise 7, 9, 14 or 21 breaths, with a Cleansing Breath between each cycle (pages 87–8).

Quiet Recharging Cycle

In this cycle, inhaling and exhaling is done through the nose. Each exercise is practised standing straight, with feet together.

1. Inhale a full abdominal breath. Retain the breath by closing the glottis (as though swallowing).
   Hold the breath as long as you comfortably can; then breathe out, concentrating on the thought that you are directing the *prana* to the solar plexus, and exhaling only air.
2. Inhale. Slowly stretch your arms forward and clench your fists as though grasping a rod. Retain the breath. Exhale, directing *prana* to solar plexus, as in (1).
3. Inhale slowly. Tense every muscle of the body. Retain breath. Then relax and exhale, directing *prana* to the solar plexus.
4. Inhale. Rise up on the tips of the toes. Retain breath and position; then exhale, concentrating on *prana* going to solar plexus.
5. Inhale. Raise the arms, placing palms together above your head. Retain as long as comfortable, then exhale, directing *prana* as above.

*Students can learn to use this slowing of the breath in their daily life . . . helping to calm themselves when emotionally upset, nervous or harassed. When agitated the breathing rate quickens; when the breath is slowed down the agitation subsides.

6. Inhale. Retain breath with your palms pressed together before the chest, in attitude of prayer. Exhale, directing *prana* as above.
7. Inhale. Raise arms above the head, slowly bringing them down into attitude of prayer as in (6). Exhale, concentrating on solar plexus.

This *Quiet Cycle* may be performed up to three times, not more. Each group of seven breaths should be separated by a powerful cleansing breath.

Vigorous cycle

This cycle also consists of seven breaths. It differs from the quiet cycle in the vigorous movements of the arms and in exhalation through the mouth.

All exercises are practised standing straight, with feet together.

1. Inhale a full breath. Lock it in the chest and swing the arms twice forward, twice backward in a circular movement, like windmills. Exhale through the mouth.
2. Stretch both arms forward. Inhale. Retaining breath, and keeping arms at shoulder level, bring back to the sides, then together again, two or three times vigorously. Exhale.
3. Inhale, swinging arms up and slightly back over the head, arching the back. Repeat two or three times, then exhale.
4. Inhale. Raise arms and join hands over head. Bend body once to the right side, once to left, bending from the waist. Exhale.
5. Inhale slowly. Stretch both arms forward, and while retaining breath, bring them back towards you two or three times vigorously (as though pulling back), shaking the whole body. Exhale.
6. Inhale. Retain the breath and place the palms on the ribs. Vigorously massage and squeeze the floating ribs. Exhale.
7. Inhale, retain the breath and gently tap the chest with the fingers as you exhale.

In all these exercises the mind is concentrated on the solar plexus, forming the image of *prana* retained there, while the stale air and tiredness are expelled with vigorous exhalation.

Conclude the cycle with the traditional cleansing breath.

83

Great Physical breath of a yogi

This consists of four deep breaths and prolonged retention (as long as comfortable) with the mind concentrated alternatively on the head, the heart, the stomach and the spine ... the four most vital parts of the body.

All the breaths are performed standing straight and with inhalation and exhalation through the nose.

1. Place the palms flat on top of the head with the fingers laced together. Inhale, and retaining breath, stretch the arms up, turning the palms upward, but still keeping fingers interlaced. Direct *prana* to the head. Exhale and relax.
2. Hands with fingers interlaced are rested on the chest. Inhale, stretch arms forward turning palms away from you, but keeping fingers laced. Send *prana* to the heart. Exhale and relax.
3. Fingers laced together, hold the hands loosely in front of the body, arms hanging down in a relaxed way. Inhale. Turn the palms down towards the ground, tensing the arms, and forming a mental image of *prana* directed to the stomach. Exhale.
4. Hands behind the back with fingers loosely laced. Inhale, stretch and tense arms downwards, turning palms towards ground. Send *prana* to the spine and exhale.

Further recharging breaths

Breath of circulating life force

1. Sitting on the floor, stretch the legs, lean forward and take hold of the big toes, using index fingers, and interlocking the thumbs (see Fig. C). Lock the chin to the chest, and deeply and rhythmically breathe in and out, with the mind concentrated on the thought of *prana* circulating within the body.

In this exercise, *prana*, flowing from the finger-tips, is directed to the legs, whence it circulates through the whole body, benefiting the vital organs.

Solar Plexus breath

Lying flat on the back with the legs loosely crossed, place your finger-tips lightly on the solar plexus. Breathe deeply and con-

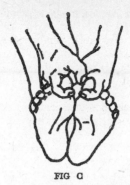

FIG C

centrate the mind on the image of life force directed to this area. The exercise could be done with the legs straight.

Breathing through the bones

"Nature's blessing is on the yogi who knows how to breathe with his bones." This quotation from an ancient treatise on breathing is not enigmatic to the student who understands breath control.

In the West we are taught that we breathe with the skin, but yoga teaches that the entire body, including the vital organs and bones, can be trained to participate in the act of breathing. The method is based on the *pranic* theory that life force could be consciously directed to any part of the system by the trained adept.

Lie down on the back, completely relaxed. Concentrate on breathing in and out through the bones of the legs, through the bones of the arms, chest and skull. You must learn how to visualize this process. Draw the life force right through your body with incoming and outgoing breath.

The method is wonderfully invigorating.

Breathing away tiredness

Lying flat on the back, relaxed, establish slow deep breathing. Imagine that with each incoming breath *prana* is being drawn in, filling the whole body; and with outgoing breath you are sending it out through the millions of hair-pores of the skin.

Yoga teaches that tiredness comes from an accumulation of impurities in the body. Through this exercise you are speeding purification of the blood-stream, forcing tiredness, and impurities, out through the pores.

Breath directed to the spine
Athletes, sportsmen, bushwalkers, know the invigorating effect of a shower after a strenuous day. The stream of hot water pouring down the spine literally washes away tiredness.

The same and even more profound benefit can be achieved by sending *prana* to the spine, while lying completely relaxed. With each calm and deep *exhalation* the roots of the spinal nerves are warmed up and refreshed.

Breathing cycle practised lying on the floor
Inhale and exhale through the nose.

1. Lie on the back with the arms stretched over the head. Inhale, stretching arms and tensing whole body. Exhale and relax.
2. Inhale, lifting the chest only. Exhale and relax.
3. Inhale, lifting only hips. Exhale and relax.
4. Inhale, bring the knees up to the stomach, pressing them against the solar plexus with the hands. Exhale and relax.

Increasing vital energy through the elements

"I am in everything, and everything is in me."

In modern terms this could be explained as diffusing macrocosm and microcosm. Yoga takes it literally, transferring life force from the elements to the human body, to strengthen and increase its vital energy. In this cycle, the recharging medium is the breath, and the *prana* or life force is drawn from the Sun, Earth, Air and Water.

Energy from the Sun
This is one of the oldest techniques of *Hatha* yoga.

Sit facing the sun, wearing as little clothing as possible. Establish rhythmical breath and concentrate on the thought that with *inhalation* you are drawing in the energy of the sun, with *exhalation* transforming it into your own energy.

It is most effective done early in the morning before the sun is too strong. Turn your body 90 degrees at intervals of five minutes (or longer if the sun is not too hot) so that you finally complete a circle and the whole body is sunned.

An ancient "sun stone" for this purpose was used by Michael Volin in a Chinese *ashram*. Set in the centre of the inner court-yard, it was a flat, circular stone, about three feet in diameter, resting horizontally on an upright base. The yogi recharging himself by sun sat on it while another disciple turned it 90 degrees every five minutes or so.

Energy from the Earth
Sit with the legs crossed, in a quiet and secluded place in the open, in the shade. Rest the hands on the knees with thumb and index fingers closed in the traditional position, and the rest of the fingers stretched down to make contact with the earth. (If you cannot get your knees down close enough to the earth and your fingers are not touching it, stretch the arms out at the sides of the thighs. The main object is to touch the earth with the finger-tips.)

Establish deep breathing and concentrate the mind on the thought of drawing the energy of Mother Earth through your finger-tips with *incoming breath*, and with *exhalation* transferring it to your own energy.

Energy from the Air
Sit with the legs crossed, in the open, and establish deep breath-ing. Raise your arms over your head, holding them parallel and with palms facing. The fingers should be stretched and apart. (The hands are acting as antennae.)

Imagine that the energy of the Ether or Air is entering your finger-tips with each *inhalation* and with *each outgoing breath* is transferred to yourself.

Energy from the Water
This is practised while floating in the water. Rhythmical breathing is established and as you *inhale* you absorb the energy of the water through the pores; as you *exhale* you transfer it to yourself.

Purifying Breaths

Blacksmith's Bellows. (*Bhastrica*)
Sitting in the cross-legged position, breathe in and out through the nostrils about ten times, quickly and deeply, like an athlete who has just finished a strenuous run.

Then inhale a deep breath and forming the lips into an O,

exhale in short sharp bursts until the lungs are completely empty.

Repeat two or three times.

The exercise is very powerful and is known as the "Bloodstream purifier". Oxygen is literally pumped into the bloodstream, as a blacksmith's bellows blow air into the fire to make it burn more brightly.

A variation is to inhale and exhale through alternative nostrils. After practice it is advisable to wash out the nostrils with warm salted water.

Cleansing or HA Breath

This is a very important part of breathing practice and must be learnt correctly.

There are two main kinds of cleansing breaths described in Indian yoga; and Chinese breathing gymnastics (which possibly stemmed from yoga) describes an additional one.

With the feet apart, slowly inhale a full breath, raising the arms up from the sides till they are stretched over the head. Then vigorously throw the top part of the body forward (keeping the legs straight), at the same time exhaling through the mouth with the sound "Ha". Imagine that you are not only getting rid of the stale air in the lungs, but every trace of tiredness.

Practise three times.

Standing Cleansing Breath

Stand straight and slowly inhale full breath; then forming an O with the lips, vigorously exhale in a series of sharp blasts, rapidly contracting the floating ribs and diaphragm.

In Chinese breathing gymnastics, the air is expelled in this manner, accompanied by rubbing the lower ribs, and by tapping the chest.

The Cleansing Breath is taken from nature. Every day millions of tired people unconsciously perform a cleansing breath when they sigh. A sigh is a kind of safety valve which relieves accumulated tension, but the yoga cleansing breath is much more powerful, and is also accompanied by *concentration on the idea of expelling all tiredness*, as well as stale air.

The permanent presence of stale air in the lungs is responsible for many vague feelings of malaise, the headaches, lethargy, sluggishness, and loss of vitality which so many people endure.

Cooling and Warming Breaths

Physical yoga has been practised for centuries in both hot and cold parts of the East, and has a number of techniques designed to combat the effects of temperature and give the yogi power over the elements.

All cooling and warming methods are a combination of breathing and concentration; and they are based on the belief that *prana*, being a cosmic energy, can be transformed into the sensation of heat or cold.

1. *Cooling Breath*

Sit with the legs crossed. Establish deep breathing and imagine that with each *exhalation* you are transforming *prana* into a pleasant sensation of coolness. Concentrate either upon the whole body, or on the spine which will eventually lead to the same sensation.

2. *Breathing through a Crow's Beak*

Sitting cross-legged, close the mouth except for a tiny opening. Inhale through this "crow's beak" opening, with a hissing sound, keeping the tongue close to the lips. Exhale slowly through the nose.

This breath creates a pleasant cooling sensation in the mouth, which gradually spreads all over the body. It also has the power to appease thirst.

Warming Breath

Many travellers in North China, the Himalayas, Tibet have been astonished to see yogis sitting in the snow, in a temperature below zero, wearing only a loin-cloth; or standing on a mountain peak in a blizzard, sometimes for hours, without any ill effects.

In these parts of the world the ability to defy cold has become an art, and is a challenge to an adept.

Warming Breath is based on the same principle as Cooling Breath. The yogi converts *prana* into a sensation of bodily warmth with his outgoing breath, concentrating on the *absolute belief* that he will succeed.

In Michael Volin's Sydney yoga school there are many students who have mastered this technique well enough to be able to enjoy surfing all the year round.

Sit with the legs crossed.

Establish breath and start by concentrating on a small area of the body . . . the middle of the palm or the index finger . . . creating in it a sensation of warmth.

Only after you have succeeded in this one spot can you start to enlarge the field of concentration, gradually warming the whole hand, arm, back.

In winter the feet could be warmed in this way, which is healthier than using a hot water bottle.

Do not be discouraged if you do not succeed at once. It is not easy and you must persevere. You must develop an intense ability to concentrate; also a different attitude to cold, for self-hypnosis is an important part of the exercise. One student actually produced a blister in the middle of her palm as a result of her concentration.

Pacifying Breaths

Cycle of tranquillizing breaths

One of the most efficient ways to pacify the mind and nervous system is through the practice of nine extremely slow breaths, known as the *Pacifying Cycle*.

The breathing is done in the standing position, with feet together, and the arms slowly moving. Inhaling and exhaling is through the nose.

For the first four breaths, bring the arms slowly forward, and upward, joining them over the head. Then lower them at the sides as you exhale.

In the next three breaths the arms are raised from the sides to join over the head, with inhalation, and lowered to the sides with exhalation.

For the last two breaths arms are raised forward (holding them parallel) and above the head while inhaling, and brought down in the same way during exhalation.

During the first four breaths concentrate the mind on a circle.
During the second three breaths concentrate on a triangle.
During the last two breaths concentrate on parallel lines.

OM Breath

This is one of the yogi's most beautiful pacifying breaths.

Sit in one of the cross-legged poses. Inhale, and retain the breath, concentrating the mind on the sound OM for a second or two, then exhale.

The syllable *OM*, "mother of all sounds", silently vibrating in the mind, brings great calmness and tranquillity.

Directing prana to others

Prana may be directed to others, either by direct contact or from a distance.

In the direct contact method the two practitioners sit face to face, with their feet placed together, holding each other's hands and both deeply breathing.

With the outgoing breath of the sender, the receiver should inhale, concentrating on the thought of absorbing life force.

There is some danger in this practice, for the sender could easily drain off his own life force, leaving himself defenceless. After every few breaths he must perform some recharging techniques himself.

It is also believed that *prana* could be sent through space, no matter what distance, just as it is sent by direct contact. It is equally beneficial with or without the knowledge of the receiver.

The image of the receiver must be evoked by the sender.

Breathing away pain

In sitting pose or lying on the back, establish slow breathing and concentrate on directing life force to the seat of the pain. The mind must be fixed on the thought of Breathing away Pain.

Take half a tumbler of cool water just before practising this exercise, which is used for headaches, backaches, toothache, etc

9

PRELIMINARY EXERCISES, LIMBERING-UP MOVEMENTS, EXERCISES FOR CIRCULATION AND TO FIRM-UP FLESH AND MUSCLES

The flabby flesh and sagging muscles so common in middle-age usually come from lack of exercise and/or loss of weight. They are depressing reminders of passing time, but may be improved by regular practice of the movements given in this chapter.

These exercises are part of a series known as the Magic of Slow Movements, which are also used for body-building and body-moulding in yoga training. They are very effective if practised with absolute regularity and full mental concentration. They should be done in front of a looking-glass, or with the eyes shut, picturing the body as you wish it to be.

Perform each movement four times.

You will soon learn to identify the different sets of muscles you are working on and can then direct your mind to each one in turn, encouraging it to respond, willing it to regain its former strength and elasticity. The constructive power of the mind is a most important part of the Slow Movements.

This chapter also includes other exercises for improving different parts of the body; a series for limbering-up, and another for improving circulation.

Limbering-up movements

Limbering-up should always be done before yoga practice, as dancers warm up their muscles.

1. Start with the shoulders, bringing them both forward in a hunching movement, then back and again forward, continuously, without jerking or pausing. After three or four such movements reverse the action, both shoulders going back; and finally rotate each shoulder separately, as though swimming backstroke, letting one shoulder come forward as the other goes back and pivoting the spinal vertebrae one upon the other in their sockets.

Although the movement is done with shoulders and arms, the exercise is really designed to keep the spine supple and to send extra blood to the roots of the spinal nerves. When practised correctly it brings a very pleasant glowing sensation in the back and between the shoulder-blades, particularly to one who has been sitting all day at a desk.

2. Standing with feet apart, stretch up your arms as high as you can, as though trying to touch the ceiling; then let yourself fall forward from the waist, hands brushing the floor. Stretching upward, the muscles should be tensed; in falling forward they should be completely relaxed . . . head lolling, arms dangling like a rag doll.

   This is not only a good exercise for muscles and waistline but is a study of complete muscular relaxation; a way of learning to let go.

3. Let the top part of your body, from the waist, fall limply, in the same way, over to the left, then forward. Come up, fall to the right, then forward. Come up and repeat to the left, then the right; and finally try to let it go back, bending at the waistline, putting pressure on the small of the back. Let your head fall back as limply and relaxed as possible.

4. Rotate your whole body, starting with the head. Move it round in a circle, to the left; then circle the shoulders, then the chest, then from the waistline with the hands brushing the floor. Come up, wait a moment, then repeat the process in the opposite direction. All the movements must be limp, without any muscles tensed.

   Students often start by *bending* down, which is quite a different thing and quite wrong. If you can remember that this is a relaxing exercise it may help to get it right.

   These forward-falling movements are prohibited for people with hypertension, since they bring blood to the head; but for this reason they are excellent rejuvenators, helping delay wrinkles through feeding the facial tissues with extra arterial blood.

Cycle to improve circulation

These exercises improve the circulation and overcome cold hands and feet, chilblains and cramp. In winter they should be practised regularly every morning and evening, and during the day if necessary. The foot and ankle exercises also strengthen calf and ankle muscles.

93

1. *For the arms*. Stretch the arms out at the sides and circle them with fluttering movements, as a child does when pretending to fly or playing fairies. Continue the movements for a few seconds, letting the hands flutter as well.
2. Now shake your hands, vigorously, away from your body, from the wrists, as though shaking off water.
3. Separate your fingers, and, keeping them slightly bent, move them individually as though playing scales or five-anger exercises on the air.
4. Standing with hands on your hips, kick out with the left leg, from the knee, sharply as though shaking something off your foot. Repeat with the right leg; then again with the left; then right again.
5. Standing with hands still on hips, raise right leg slightly in front and move the foot up and down from the ankle several times; then repeat with the left foot.
6. With left leg raised, circle the foot, from the ankle, several times one way, then reverse. Repeat with the right foot.
7. With feet slightly apart, swing both arms round to the right, then to the left, almost wrapping them round yourself. They should be as limp as empty sleeves.
8. Finish by falling forward from the waist, as above (number 2 – Limbering-up), then stretch up as high as you can. Relax and let yourself fall to the ground, taking care not to hurt yourself as you come down.

For the spine

To stretch and compress the spine

Stand erect with feet together and arms by the sides. Without moving a limb, try to make yourself taller, stretching the spine a fraction at a time, growing straighter and straighter, and higher and higher. (Not just raising the shoulders but really stretching the spine.)

Then begin to come down, compressing the spine, trying to make yourself smaller and smaller (but not bending the knees).

Repeat stretching again, then compressing, several times.

In young people this is recommended to encourage growth but in those who are older it is even more important in preventing shrinking and stooping.

Small of the back

Lie on your back with ankles crossed and drawn up against the stomach, and arms clasped round them. Curve your spine so that the small of the back makes contact with the floor and rock gently from side to side, as though in a cradle. This very soothing exercise is usually practised after Cobra and Locust *asanas* but may be used any time.

Rocking

This spinal massage is recommended, in conjunction with Pose of Tranquillity (page 111) for helping to overcome insomnia. It not only massages the spine but benefits the roots of the spinal nerves and soothes a nervous centre in the back of the head.

Sit with knees drawn up and hands under the thighs. Rock yourself right back, letting your feet come over your head till they touch the floor, then forward with your head between your knees; then back again, then forward, like a rocking chair, smoothly as possible without jerking.

Then cross the ankles, take hold of the toes and continue the movement.

Exercises for the stomach

1. Sit on the floor with legs stretched out in front. Put your hands on your knees and slowly lower your body till you are lying on your back, with hands flat on your thighs. Then start to sit up again, slowly, sliding the hands along the legs till they are on the knees again. Repeat three times.

   The feet must stay on the floor all the time. They must not be lifted an inch. All lowering and raising of the body is done with the stomach muscles.

2. The same exercise with the arms folded on the chest.
3. The same again with the hands clasped behind the head.

   With each changed position of the hands the exercise becomes harder. If you can master the first three movements, try to do it with the hands crossed behind your back, with both elbows rising above your head.

4. Lie on your back, then prop yourself up with your elbows with legs stretched out in front. Slowly raise and lower legs in a scissors movement, not bringing the feet down to the

ground at all and letting the stomach feel the stress. (Fig. 1.)
Repeat 3–4 times.

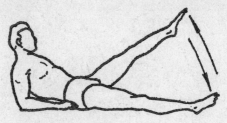

FIG 1

5. In the same position, keeping legs straight, cross and re-cross in horizontal scissors movement, 3–4 times.
6. In same position, with knees straight, separate legs and describe circles, out, up, across and then down together, then separating to circle again. Do not bring legs down to the floor between movements. (Fig. 2).

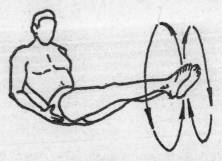

FIG 2

7. Lie on back, with knees bent and feet on floor. Sit up suddenly and stretch legs out diagonally into the air at angle of 45 degrees from floor. Lie back and relax. Repeat several times. (Fig. 3.)
8. Lie on back with hands on hips. Kick up right leg, kick higher and sit up – without support of hands – then lie back. Repeat with left leg. Repeat each side several times, then relax. (Fig. 4.)
9. Rowing. Sit up with knees bent. Lean forward, extend arms

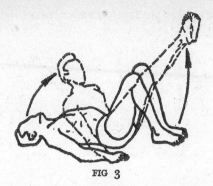

FIG 3

between knees, then pull back, stretching legs and stomach muscles. (Fig. 5.)

10. Sit up with arms folded on chest and legs stretched out in front. Swing the body over to the right, lowering it so that you are rolling on the floor but with back arched, then sit

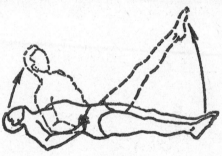

FIG 4

up quickly. Roll over to the other side, then sit up quickly. Repeat several times. This exercise is also recommended for slimming hips, thighs and waistline. (Fig. 6.)

12. Stand up with feet apart. Stretch arms forward with fists closed and turned so that the thumbs are inside, facing each other. Keeping the arms straight, slowly move them apart as though pulling a heavy spring; and at the same time lean backwards so the stomach muscles are tensed.

13. Stand with feet slightly apart. Tense the abdominal muscles until they are quite firm, then relax. Tense again and relax; tense and relax several times.

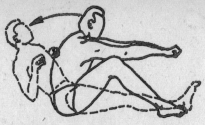

FIG 5

14. In same position, bend down and pick up an imaginary bar-bell. Lift it without bending the knees, so that the stomach muscles do the work.
15. In the same position, stretch the arms forward and raise the same imaginary bar-bell up over your head without bending the elbows. Repeat several times.
16. Lie on your back. Draw the knees up to the stomach, stretch them up at right angles to the body, then slowly lower them, controlling the movement with the muscles of the stomach.

Asanas which will help improve your stomach muscles are: *Uddiyana* (page 124); *Nauli* (page 151); Bow Pose (Appendix); Cobra (page 121); Locust (page 122); Plough (page 119); Archer (page 120); Spinal Twist (page 120); Supine Pelvic (page 150); Head-to-Knee (page 120) and all forward stretching cycles (pages 118–120).

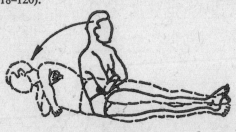

FIG 6

For waist and hips

Waist

1. Stand with feet together and arms by sides. Imagine you are

98

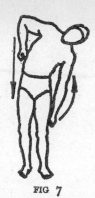

FIG 7

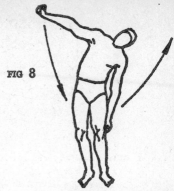

FIG 8

lifting a heavy weight with your left hand and that you must keep your hand close to your side as you do so. The fist, which is clenched, should just about brush your side as it travels up into the armpit. Relax and repeat with the other side. (Fig. 7.)

2. Repeat movement with feet apart.
3. Standing with arms by sides, raise right arm, slowly, as though you can hardly prise it away from your side. Lower it and repeat with left arm. (Fig. 8.)
4. Repeat with feet apart.
5. Stand with legs apart and arms stretched out at sides. Bend forward, twisting body so that right palm is *flat* on the floor beside left foot. Come up and repeat on the other side. (Fig. 9.) Do not bend the knees.

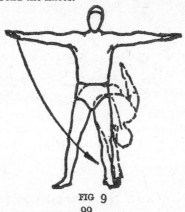

FIG 9

6. Standing in same position, but with hands on the back of thighs. Bend forward, sliding hands down back of legs, take hold of ankles and try to press head first to left knee, then to right knee. Come up, and repeat several times. Do not bend knees.

7. Stand with feet apart and arms stretched over head. Clasp your hands, then lean over to right side, then up, then to left side, then up. Keep the body straight and do not bend forward. Repeat several times, then relax.

8. In same position, clasp hands and twist body, from waistline only, first to right, then to left, keeping feet flat on the floor. Also practice the following exercises in the stomach series: Numbers 5–10, and 12. Vary Number 12 in stomach exercises (pulling open heavy spring) by turning first to the right side, then to the left, as you move the arms. Be sure you twist only from the waist. (Fig. 10.)

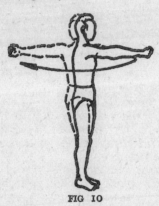

FIG 10

Asanas that will improve the waistline are: Spinal Twist (page 120); Sideways Swing (page 121); Head-to-Knee (page 120); Forward stretching (pages 118–19).

Hips

1. Sit on the floor with legs stretched out in front. Put hands on your hips and thrust legs forward, first left, then right, actually walking on the buttocks. After several movements, reverse, walking backwards in the same way.

2. Lie on your back with knees bent and soles of feet on floor. Swing hips and legs from side to side, twisting from the waistline, keeping the top part of the body still and legs together. Bring legs over till they touch the floor each side, massaging the hips in the process. (Fig. 11.) Bend both knees.

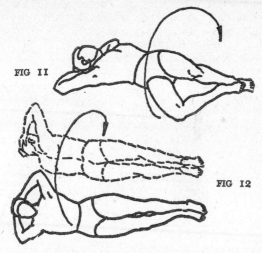

FIG 11

FIG 12

3. Lie on the floor with your hands clasped on top of your head. Roll right over to one side, arching your back and keeping the body stiff, then over to the other side, putting all the weight on the hips. (Fig. 12.)
4. Lie on your back, then prop yourself up on your elbows as in stomach exercise Number 4. Raise left leg, bend the knee and circle the leg out and round several times, with toe pointed, stretching leg as you bring it back alongside right leg. Then repeat process with the right leg. (Fig. 13.)

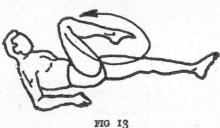

FIG 13

5. Same as Number 3, exercise for thighs.
6. Same as Number 10 for stomach.
7. Sit back on heels with arms linked over head. Slide body from heels to floor, on right side, arching your body to the left; then slide across heels again and come down on the left side, arching the body to the right. Continue moving from one side to the other, massaging hips and stretching waistline in the process.

Practise the following *asanas*: Spinal Twist (page 120); Sideways Swing (page 121); Archer (page 120); Bow (Appendix); Plough (page 119); Head-to-Knee (page 120); Cross-legged Poses (page 112) and Forward Stretching (page 118).

For the bust and chest

1. Stand with feet together. Raise the arms and grasp an imaginary rope, pulling down on it so that the chest muscles are tensed. Relax and repeat four times.
2. In same position raise arms from sides and bring them forward, with elbow straight, as if pressing down against the air, and tensing chest muscles. At about waist level, relax the pressure and start to bring the arms up again, from the sides, then pressing down again. (Fig. 14.)
3. Standing with feet together and arms at the sides. Clench fists,

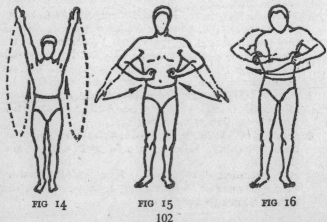

FIG 14   FIG 15   FIG 16

move arms out from sides then bring them in together, tensing chest muscles, till fists meet in front of body. Relax and repeat.

4. Repeat movement but bring arms in till fists cross in front of body.
5. This time raise the arms out at the sides. Bring the fists in, bending the elbows and keeping them held out from the body at chest level. Bring fists together in front of body in line with elbows. (Fig. 15.)
6. Start from position in which you just finished . . . elbows out from sides, fists together in front of chest. Slowly pull the fists apart as though pulling a heavy spring. Relax and repeat four times.
7. Same as Number 14 for stomach.
8. Same as Number 15 for stomach.
9. Stand with feet slightly apart, with hands clasped (palms together) in front at chest level. Push the right hand against the left, *resisting* with the left but moving both hands to the left, tensing chest muscles. Repeat same movements on the right side. (Fig. 16.)

Asanas for improving the chest and bust are: Cobra (page 121); Bow (Appendix); Head of a Cow (page 116); Pose of a Camel (page 122).

Legs, thighs and calves

1. Stand with legs apart. With hands on hips and keeping soles of feet flat on floor, bring the knees in slowly together, till they touch, then apart; together-apart; together-apart.
2. Stand with legs together. Raise right knee, and keeping thigh at right angles to the body, swing the lower leg in and out briskly several times. Lower leg and repeat with left.
3. In same position, raise knee as before, then swing it to the side, then forward . . . to side . . . forward . . . several times. Lower leg and repeat with other leg.
4. Standing with feet together, raise the toes only, then lower them; raise them, lower them and repeat several times. (Fig. 17.)
5. With feet together and hands on hips, practise stationary walking, coming on to the ball of the foot each time and arching the instep as you move.

103

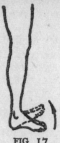

FIG 17

6. With feet together and hands on hips. Rise on to the ball of the foot, then the toes; hold a few seconds, then come down and repeat, until the legs feel tired.
7. With feet together and hands on thighs, bend knees and come down into a half-squatting position and then up again rather quickly. It should be a continuous slightly springy movement. Repeat several times.
8. With feet apart and arms stretched forward and parallel. Slowly come down into a position as though you were sitting on an invisible chair. You must keep the knees together, back perfectly straight, not leaning forward, and the soles flat on the floor. Come up and repeat. (Fig. 18.)
9. In same position, come down as before but into a squatting position, making sure the soles of the feet remain flat on the floor. The arms stretched forward should help to balance. Come up and repeat several times. (Fig. 18.)

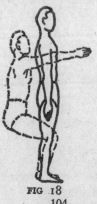

FIG 18

10. Practise circulation exercise Number 5.
11. Practise circulation exercise Number 6.

Asanas for firming the thighs: Bow (Appendix 152); Locust (page 122); Supine Pelvic (page 150); Star Pose – for inside the thighs (page 119); Variation of Head-to-Knee, with legs apart – for inside the thighs (page 120); Eagle Pose, for legs (page 117).

For arms, back and shoulders

1. *Arms.* Stand with arms by sides. Close your fists and bring them up and forward in a scooping movement, flexing biceps and triceps, bending the elbows but keeping them close to the sides. Lower arms and repeat several times.
2. Stand with arms stretched out at sides with palms facing up. Keeping arms in position, twist them so that the palms face down, round and up again, reversing movement. Do not bend the elbows. (Fig. 19.)

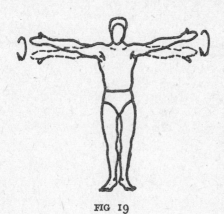

FIG 19

Shoulders and back
3. Put finger-tips on shoulders, then bring the points of the elbows together in front of your chest. Separate them, and bring them together again and repeat several times.
4. Raise the arms in front of chest with elbows bent and with clenched fists close together. Slowly move the fists apart and backwards, as though opening a heavy spring, squeezing

shoulder-blades together, putting pressure on spine and flushing roots of spinal nerves with blood. Repeat four times. See Number 5 – Bust Exercises.

5. Stand with your elbows bent, forming a V on each side of your chest. Push the hands out from the body, as though pushing against the air, in an undulating movement, downwards, outwards, and upwards, squeezing the shoulder-blades together with each movement. Repeat four times.

6. Stretch the arms out at the sides, keeping elbows straight. Raise arms over the head with palms facing downwards and tensing the muscles, then lower to shoulder level again and repeat four times.

7. With arms stretched at sides, as above, rotate them in small circles, first in forward movement, then backwards. Do not bend elbows. Repeat four times.

8. Stand erect with hands behind back, one hand clasping the other wrist. Slowly move hands up the back, flexing back muscles, then relax, lower hands and start again. Repeat four times.

It is advisable to finalize cycle of body moulding exercises with "the whole of the body" tension-relaxation movement.

Standing erect, slowly tense *every* muscle of body, inhaling and projecting the image of yourself into the future – firm, straight, youthful, unchanged. Yoga emphasizes that to achieve the full benefit of this exercise you *must* bring together the three powers – gesture, breath and mind.

10

ASANAS

In practising these exercises and *asanas* readers must use their commonsense and knowledge of their own bodies. It would be foolish for a woman of seventy, who has not exercised for forty years, to force her legs into the Lotus position, or for an overweight man with blood-pressure to stand on his head. Though there are people in their seventies who stand on their heads and perform advanced poses, others can manage quite well with substitutes or modifications, such as suggested in the following pages.

Study the pictures carefully before attempting anything. Never force or strain the body. Any sign of pain must be taken as a stop signal and the movement not attempted again until you have rested. Everything should be done slowly and cautiously, with plenty of time for relaxation; and if you find your heart beating a little fast after exertion, lie down and practise deep breathing until it quietens.

Remember that the constructive power of the mind must be brought to bear on all physical movements, whether breathing, body-building exercises or static postures.

The benefits attributed to the postures are based on traditional yoga literature, supported by many factual cases among western students. It is taught that with each *asana* mastered the body experiences a rebirth.

It is always advisable for people over forty to have a medical check-up before starting physical yoga, to ensure that there is nothing to forbid certain *asanas*.

Savasana. Pose of Complete Rest
Benefits: Complete relaxation of entire body, muscles, nerves and mind, with all attendant benefits.

Although this *asana* is performed lying flat on the floor, without moving, it is one of the hardest of all to master, for the student must learn to relax not only muscles but nerves and mind. When the technique is achieved it can bring complete rest and refreshment in a few minutes. It is an essential remedy for those suffering from hypertension, heart or nervous troubles, insomnia ... or even just the usual stress and tension of a city life. It is especially important for older people and could be practised by anyone, even a bed-ridden invalid. It is one of yoga's greatest gifts to the West – the secret of relaxation.

The exercise is done in four stages. (If possible darken the room.)

1. Lie down on the floor, on your back, and shut your eyes. Arms are by your sides and feet slightly apart. Start by relaxing the muscles, working up from the tips of the toes to the head . . . relaxing feet, ankles, calves, knees, thighs, stomach muscles; then the muscles of the waist, chest and shoulders, arms and hands. Relax the face. Let the lower jaw sag; try to relax your tongue; roll your eyes back under the closed lids; smooth out your forehead.

   If it is difficult to start this muscular relaxation, try inhaling, tensing the whole body, then exhaling and relaxing. Do this a couple of times.

   With practice you will learn to relax every single muscle, gradually *inducing* your body to become limp and lifeless. (*Savasana* means Corpse Pose, or Pose of a Dead Man.)

2. When the muscles are all relaxed, relax the nerves. Start by turning your Mind's Eye in on yourself (see exercise on page 137), trying to find the pockets of inner tension. Inner tension is quite different from muscular tension, far more destructive and harder to relax. This part of the exercise is called Withdrawal of Nervous Energy, and it should be a real withdrawal, a closing down of all the communications coming and going between nerves and brain, an ebbing away, like a tide going out, an emptying of the nervous channels. Try to think that nothing matters, that you have completely let go; that your body is growing heavier and heavier, your limbs are leaden, you could not even lift a finger, that you are sinking down into the darkness, as though going off to sleep.

3. Practise the full yoga abdominal breath, slowing down the rate of breathing (see page 81). The slow tempo, which is about five heartbeats to each inhalation, five to each exhalation, will help you to relax further. Remember that slowing the breath slows down the heart and rhythm of the whole body, pacifying the nervous centres.

   Let the stomach come out as you inhale and let it fall back as you exhale; and concentrate on the thought that with each inhalation you are taking in *prana* (see page 21) with the air,

108

and with each exhalation you are sending it all over your body, recharging yourself with vital energy.

4. Try to detach your mind and send it as far away as you can from your normal life and surroundings, leaving behind all your worries, work, responsibilities. Enter your own mental *ashram* (hermitage) (see page 134), and try to *be* there completely, leaving only your body lying on the floor. This is known as Small Exit from the Physical Body, and when properly performed completely relaxes the mind.

In the very last stage, switch off all thoughts and pictures and try to keep the mind blank (see page 136). When you finally achieve this you will know absolute relaxation of body and mind and will feel entirely recharged and refreshed.

Nervous people, ill people, harassed and overworked people should all learn this wonderful exercise. Even if practised only for five minutes a day, this is enough to recharge the body. It is also the way to overcome fatigue, to preserve vital energy, and to hold off old age.

Savasana usually comes before and after a lesson, but may be done at any time. When you finally finish the exercise, stretch and yawn before you stand up, just as you would on waking in the morning.

*Relaxing on the side**
A very pleasant exercise for the weak or elderly is to practise full abdominal breathing lying on the side. (This is one of the sleeping positions . . . see page 65.) Lie on the right side with the right arm stretched out under the head and the right knee drawn up under you. Let your left arm lie limply behind you. Inhale and exhale deeply and rhythmically for as long as you like; then turn on the other side.

Inverted Poses
With the exception of the Headstand, inverted poses are usually practised after *Savasana*, the breathing cycles and limbering-up exercises, when the body has been prepared by relaxation and warming-up.

*The system of Chinese breathing gymnastic recommends four breathing poses for sick and convalescent patients: cross-legged position; lying on the back, on the right side and on the left side, spending equal time in each.

Older students should follow this order, which minimizes any strain.

The inverted positions are among the most important of all *asanas*. When practised with full mental concentration their power is doubled.

Shoulderstand or Candle Position (Plate I)
Benefits: Delays ageing. Tones up endocrinal glands. Corrects weight. Improves varicose veins, swollen feet and ankles, thyroid deficiency, loss of energy, sexual debility, menstrual irregularity, hot flushes, displaced organs, impotence.

Lying on your back, try to raise your legs up into the position shown in the illustration. If you are stiff or overweight you will not be able to get up very far, but do the best you can, if necessary propping yourself up against the wall. Although it is desirable to perform the *asana* correctly, the main objective is to invert the body so that the legs are drained of blood.

Prop yourself up with your hands, placing them in the region of the shoulder-blades. Press your chin against your chest, shut your eyes and deeply inhale and exhale. The pressure of the chin against the chest is essential, for it is through this that the main effects of the position are achieved. The arterial blood, drained from the raised legs, flows through the rest of the body to the thyroid and para-thyroids. Since the thyroid affects all other glands the whole endocrinal system benefits.

The position should be held as long as comfortably possible, and the mind concentrated on the thought that it is a powerful tonic for the entire body; that not only the glands but every vital organ, nervous centre and muscle is being toned-up and invigorated. It is said that after the Headstand, the Candle Position is the most powerful *asana* in delaying the ageing of the body, and must be included in the daily practice. The pose produces a bio-chemical reaction and releases a latent power of self-healing, and mental concentration should direct this power to wherever it is most needed. In the East it is used as a healing pose for many maladies considered incurable by orthodox methods.

To complete the *asana*, try to bring the legs down over the head, keeping the knees straight and, if possible, touch the floor with the toes. Put the hands flat on the floor behind you to steady yourself in this position. Now concentrate your mind upon your spine and the roots of the spinal nerves, which are receiving an extra supply of arterial blood. Continue the rhythmical breathing; then bend the knees and slowly come down and relax.

Do not be discouraged if you cannot do the movements properly at first. The body will loosen up and grow stronger with practice.

Half-Shoulderstand or Half-Candle (Plate 2)
Benefits: Prevents and destroys wrinkles. Tones up skin of the face. Stimulates glands and nervous centres in the brain.

Come up into the inverted position with the legs over the head, but this time support yourself by holding your hips. Keep the elbows close to the sides, with the legs straight and the body at an angle of 45 degrees (see illustration). The chin is *not* pressed to the chest in this *asana* for its object is to send the extra blood to the face, to nourish the facial tissues.

While holding the pose, deeply inhale and exhale, with the face relaxed and the mind concentrated on the picture of yourself, forever youthful, unchangeable for years to come. This method of practice also combines the three powers – power of mind, power of breath and power of bodily position.

Hold the pose as long as you comfortably can, until you feel the pleasant warmth and fullness in the face that means the blood has reached the facial tissues; then bring the legs down over the head again, bending your knees and taking hold of your toes. Pull the legs out straight, if possible touching the toes to the floor. Let go, lower the legs and arms again, and relax.

Caution. Half-Candle is not to be practised by anyone suffering from hypertension.

Pose of Tranquillity (Triangular Pose (Plate 3)
Benefits: Promotes healthy and natural sleep, and soothes entire nervous system. Improves circulation.

Many of our students claim that when practised regularly before bedtime, this *asana* has cured them of insomnia and helped them give up sleeping pills. It is also recommended for anyone suffering from cold feet.

It is a little more difficult in the beginning than the two preceding inverted *asanas* for it is partly a balancing pose. Lying on the floor, start by stretching your arms above your head, then raise your legs and try to bring them right over the head until they form an angle of 45 degrees with the body (see illustration). Raise the arms, keeping the elbows stiff, and rest the legs on the palms of the hands. The arms form the third side of the triangle.

The body should be locked firmly and comfortably in this position. The actual position of the hands on the legs varies according to the individual length of the students' arms and legs and can only be found by experimenting. You could prop yourself up against the wall while you try to find the right position.

When you have mastered the pose, hold it as long as you can, with eyes closed, deeply breathing in and out, and mind concentrated on the thought of peace. After a short time there is often an actual sensation of drowsiness.

Choking Pose (*Plate* 4)

The Pose following the above *asana* may be a little strenuous, but for those who wish to try it, bring the legs down over the head, split the knees and press them to the floor with the hands, one on each side of the head, effecting a gentle pressure on the thyroid gland. Release the pressure, come down and relax.

Those who do not aspire to the Choking Pose should just lower the legs as in Candle or Half-Candle Poses.

After practising the Inverted Cycles it is a good idea to rest in the *Pose of a Fish* (page 121) . . . modified version. (Plate 29.)

Sitting Poses (*See also Chapter* 12, *Mental Training*)

With the exception of the Lotus Position – and possibly Pose of a Hero – the yoga sitting poses could be safely practised by anyone, of any age. They are mainly used for mental exercises, for meditation, for breathing cycles, and for eye and neck exercises.

Simple Crosslegged or Easy Pose

This is the most commonly used sitting position, in which the legs are crossed and the hands rest on the knees, or are clasped loosely in the lap, or placed one upon the other, palms uppermost. Neck and back should be held in a straight line.

Pose of an Adept (*Plate* 5)

Bring one heel close to the body, and place the other foot on the bent leg, between the thigh and calf, as shown in the illustration. Alternative sides may be used.

Half-Lotus (*Plate* 6)

Bring one heel close to the body, as above, but lift the other foot and bring it up higher, into the groin. It should actually press upon one of the arteries in this region. Alternative sides may be used.

Lotus or Buddha Pose (Plate 7)

Benefits: Develops confidence and tranquillity. Stimulates mental processes. Corrects rheumatism, constipation, indigestion.

Alternative sides may be used.

First the right foot is brought up into the left groin, as in Half-Lotus, then the left foot is lifted into the right groin, with both legs now interlocked. Hands are rested on the knees, with thumb and forefingers closed, or held in the lap, with palms open, one upon the other, as described in Easy Pose.

Caution. None of the cross-legged poses, especially Lotus and Half-Lotus, should be practised for any length of time if there are varicose veins. All these positions slow down the circulation in the legs, thus promoting blood supply to other parts of the body, with refreshing and rejuvenating effects.

It is very satisfying to be able to sit in the Lotus Position but it is not essential for the ordinary student, and if it presents great difficulties one of the easier positions should be substituted.

Diamond Pose (Plate 8)

Benefits: Strengthens knees, ankles and insteps; relieves rheumatism.

This pose, which is simple to perform, is associated with purification of the body by air. With legs together, sit back on your heels with your hands on the knees, back and head erect. Inhale through the nose, and with the eyes closed concentrate on the thought of sending *prana* or life force right through the body, directed finally through the anus.

Not to be practised for any length of time with varicose veins.

Pose of a Frog (Plate 9)

Benefits: Strengthens knees and insteps. Stimulates vital abdominal organs through movement of diaphragm breathing. Tones up genital organs.

One of the best poses in which to practice the complete abdominal breath of a yogi. Sit with the knees wide apart, toes together and weight resting on the heels. (See illustration.) Raise the hands and join the palms above the head; close the eyes, and inhale and exhale, inflating and deflating the stomach like a frog. The raised position of the hands prevents the shoulder movement typical in shallow respiration, and induces full diaphragm breathing.

A further exercise in this position is to inhale, and direct *prana* through the body with exhalation, cleansing the system with air.

The *prana* is directed finally through the genital organs, with purifying effects. See also *Aswini-mudra* (page 116).

Pose of a Child (*Plate* 10)
Benefits: Relaxes the spine and attached ligaments. Sends blood to the face and head. Tones up solar plexus.

Pose of a Child is usually practised after stretching poses.

With knees and feet together, sit back on the heels, bend forward till the forehead rests on the floor (see illustration) with arms lying limply by the sides. Inhale and exhale in a natural rhythmical way.

Pose of a Hare (*Plate* 11)
Benefits: Stimulates nervous centres and glands in the brain. Feeds facial tissues and skin of the face, teeth, ears and hair.

Although the whole body is not inverted in this pose, in a mild way it produces the same benefits as the Headstand, and is recommended for those who are not strong enough to stand on their heads.

Get into the Pose of a Child; then lean forward until the crown of the head is resting on the floor, with the back and buttocks raised. Hands are holding the ankles (see illustration). Hold as long as comfortable, inhaling and exhaling peacefully.

Pose of a Hero (*Plate* 12)
Practised with alternate legs.

Although this *asana* has some physical effects in limbering up the hips, knees and ankles, its main importance is on the spiritual plane. It is the pose assumed during concentration upon Inner Strength, and is said to develop this quality.

Sitting on the floor, bend back the right leg so that the calf is beside the body. Place the left foot high up on the right thigh, in the Half-Lotus position. The pose is held during meditation, and is accompanied by deep breathing. If Half-Lotus is too difficult, rest the sole of the left foot against the right thigh.

Pose of a Lion (*Plate* 13)
Benefits: Strengthens and improves the throat and root of tongue. Benefits facial muscles.

This pose could be practised in the open air, on a sunny day, or indoors. Sit in the Diamond Pose (page 113), facing the sun. Put your hands on your knees, straighten your back, stiffen the body and open the mouth wide. Put out the tongue as far as it will go, tilting the head so that the rays of the sun can reach down into the throat. Hold the pose for 2–3 seconds, then relax. When the body is stiffened, the fingers are also stiffened and stretched wide apart.

When done indoors, the eyes are kept open; when outdoors, facing the sun, they are closed.

Dangerous Pose (Fig. A)
Used by celibate yogis for transmuting sexual energy into physical or mental energy.

Sit with thighs crossed so that they overlap each other, with the right foot by the left side of the body and the left foot by the right side. The hands, with fingers stretched, and palms down, are placed one upon the other, on the uppermost knee. Hold the pose, inhaling and exhaling deeply, with the mind concentrated on transmuting sexual energy.

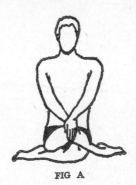

FIG A

Yoga-mudra
Benefits: Tones up abdominal and reproductive organs. Brings extra blood to the face and head, acting as a rejuvenator. Improves memory.

To perform this *asana* properly it is necessary to sit in the Lotus position, but it may also be practised in simple cross-legged pose. Put your hands behind your back with one hand holding the other wrist. Inhale; lean forward and touch the floor with the forehead. Hold the pose and breath for a few seconds, then sit up, exhale and tap the face with the finger-tips (for stimulating facial tissues).

You could vary the breathing by inhaling, exhaling as you

115

bend down, and, holding the forehead on the floor for a few seconds, with the lungs empty.

Aswini-mudra
Benefits: Stimulates nerves and organs of the reproductive system. Improves sexual debility, haemorrhoids, prolapse in women and enlarged prostate gland in men.

Sit in the Diamond Pose (page 113), Simple Cross-Legged Position, or Pose of a Frog (page 113). Inhale, exhale, and contract the muscles of the anus, drawing them inward and upward. Hold for a few seconds, then relax. Inhale, exhale again and repeat the combined exhalation-contraction, inhalation-relaxing movement. After the rhythm is mastered, practise carefully and gradually until you can do the contractions more rapidly. The exercise may be adapted to tone up the vaginal muscles in women.

Vajroli-mudra (*Plate* 14)
Benefits: Increases vital energy. Tones up solar plexus.

Sit with knees bent and drawn up, and feet flat on the floor. The palms are flat on the floor, at the sides. Inhale, and stretch the legs out at an angle of 45 degrees to the floor. Retain position, then exhale and relax.

Due to the angle of the legs in this *asana* the blood drained from them is directed to the solar plexus (the seat of energy in the body) which is toned-up and stimulated. Pressure on this plexus caused by the position of the body is also beneficial.

Head of a Cow (*Plate* 15)
Benefits: Preserves youthful appearance of the face. Firms up arms, chest and back muscles.

The pose may be performed either sitting back on the heels with the legs together (as in Diamond Pose) or on crossed ankles. The hands are locked behind the back, level with the shoulder-blades. (One arm is bent back and down over the shoulder and the other is bent up from the waistline to meet it.) (See illustration.)

Inhale and exhale while holding the pose; then bend forward and try to bring the forehead to the floor. Sit up, change the arms and repeat the movement. During the *asana* the mind should be concentrated on the rejuvenation of the face. It is said that when the right elbow is raised the left side of the face is affected, and when the left elbow is raised it affects the right side. Try to

116

influence and direct the blood to the part of your face where it is most needed.

Balancing Poses

The yoga balancing poses have a dual effect, developing not only a sense of physical balance but mental equilibrium and tranquillity; as though the physical effort of balancing the body is reflected on the mind and nervous system.

Stand on each leg in turn.

1. On the right foot, and with right hand on the hip, raise the left leg and rest the sole of the foot against the inside of the right knee, forming a triangle.

    The left hand is placed on the left knee (see Plate 16a).

2. *Tree Pose*. Bend the left leg behind you, holding the ankle, and raise the right arm in the air. (Plate 17.) Press the heel against the buttocks, arching the back slightly and raising the face to the ceiling.

3. *Variation of Tree Pose* (*Plate* 16b). Lift the left leg up on to the right thigh, as high as possible, as though you were putting it into the Half-Lotus, with the heel near the groin. The arms are raised over the head with the palms placed together. Inhale and exhale with the eyes focused on the tip of the nose. Alternatively, modify the position of the left leg as shown in the illustration.

    Each time you practise, try to hold the position a little longer until you can retain it for several minutes.

Pose of an Eagle (*Plate* 18)

As well as its effect on mental and physical balance, this *asana* strengthens the legs and ankles and, through putting pressure on the sex glands, helps to regulate menstrual irregularities, correct sterility and sexual debility.

Standing on the left foot, with the knee slightly bent, wind the other leg right round it, hooking the foot round the calf, as shown in the illustration. Then lean forward and rest the elbow on the knee, with the arms twisted in the same way as the legs, and the chin resting on the back of the hand. Hold for a few seconds with the eyes focused on the tip of the nose. Then relax, and repeat, changing legs and arms.

Angular Pose (*Plate* 19)

This is a sitting balancing pose.

Sit with the knees bent. Take hold of your big toes and slowly stretch out your legs until they are perfectly straight, and the whole body is balanced on the buttocks. Hold the pose without falling over backwards. Slow inhalation and exhalation will help in retaining the balance.

Stretching Cycle

There are many stretching *asanas*, for yoga puts the greatest emphasis on the importance of a supple spine and mobile joints. It is said that old age begins with stiffening of the backbone. Students who have passed the age of forty should pay particular attention to this cycle. Remember that nothing must be forced; that you must be content to improve a little at a time. All *asanas* are accompanied by inhalation and exhalation, and by mental concentration.

Forward Stretching
Benefits: Limbers up spine and joints. Reduces stomach and waistline. Massages abdominal organs.

Arch Gesture (*Plate* 20)
Sit with left leg stretched straight out in front and right leg bent at the knee, with the foot pressed flat against the left thigh. (See illustration.) Rest the hands on the knees. Inhale, and as you exhale, lean forward, trying to take hold of your left foot, pressing your forehead to the left knee. Do not worry if you cannot get right down, it becomes easier with practice; but do not bend the left knee, for this destroys the value of the *asana*. Repeat the movement, with inhalation and exhalation; then change legs and practise on the other side.

Variations of Arch Gesture
In each variation, one leg is stretched and the other is bent. Each changed position of the bent leg puts pressure on different parts of the abdomen as you lean forward. By practising all the variations you massage all the abdominal organs. Inhale and exhale as you bring the head down to the knee. Each movement to be practised twice on each side.

1. With right leg stretched and the left bent as in Arch Gesture, but with the foot *under* the right thigh.

118

2. With right leg stretched and left bent back so that foot and ankle are at the side of the body. Hold the left ankle with the left hand, and try to reach right foot with right hand as you come forward.
3. With right leg stretched and left knee bent and drawn up, with foot flat on the floor close to the body.
4. With right leg stretched and left leg in Half-Lotus Position. (Knee bent and flat on the floor and foot up on the right thigh, close to the groin.)
5. Sit with both legs crossed. Inhale: take hold of your toes (arms outside the knees); exhale, coming down and trying to touch the floor with your forehead. (Plate 21.)
6. With both legs stretched. Inhale: exhale, and come down trying to put hands on the toes and pressing head to the knees. (Plate 22a.)

Star Pose (Plate 23)
Benefits: Keeps spine supple. Loosens hip joints. Firms flesh inside upper thighs.

Sit with the knees wide apart, and the soles of the feet flat against each other. Hands are on the ankles. Inhale. As you exhale, take hold of your toes and try to bring your head down so that you can press them against your forehead.

This is a strenuous *asana* and should not be done more than once a day.

Plough Pose (Plate 24)
Benefits: Keeps the spine supple, corrects constipation, digestive trouble and irregular menstruation. Reduces fat on stomach.

Lie on your back with your arms by your sides. Lift your legs and try to bring them right over your head until the toes touch the floor. (This is commonly done after Candle or Shoulderstand.) Hold the pose, inhaling and exhaling; then come slowly down and relax.

An alternative position is to stretch the arms over the head and take hold of the toes as they rest on the floor, keeping the knees straight.

To stretch and exercise the spine, practise this variation:

Link the arms loosely on the floor over the head (see illustration). Bring the legs right over, as described above, and rest them with the toes flat, not dug into the floor. Move the toes to and from your head, sliding them on the floor, stretching and

119

relaxing the spine. Repeat four or five times, then come down and relax.

Head-to-Knee Pose. Standing (*Plate 22b*)

Benefits: Corrects constipation and digestive troubles. Tones up liver, kidneys and pancreas. Regulates menstruation. Reduces fat on waist and stomach.

This is the same *asana* as Number 5 on page 119 but performed in standing position. Inhale: put the hands on the backs of the thighs and as you exhale, lean forward, sliding the hands down the backs of the legs till you take hold of the ankles, and press the head against the knees. *Do not bend the knees*. Repeat once more.

Pose of an Archer (*Plate 25*)

Benefits: Loosens spine and joints; reduces fat on hips and stomach; improves vitality and digestion. Helps overcome constipation.

Sit with left leg stretched out in front. Step over it with the right leg, putting the foot flat on the floor, close to the left knee. Inhale; exhale and lean forward, putting the right hand on the toes of the left foot and taking hold of the right foot with the left hand. Try to lift this foot up and touch the big toe against the point between the eyebrows (see illustration). Remember that you are imitating the movement of an archer pulling back the string of his bow, and that the elbow (the left elbow) of the hand that is raising the foot should be held out and up, away from the body. This gives greater freedom of movement and makes the *asana* easier to perform, apart from its aesthetic value.

Change legs and arms and repeat.

Little Twist (*Plate 26*)

Benefits: Exercises spine, stimulates adrenal glands and reduces stomach and waistline.

Sit in the *Pose of an Archer* described above, with the hands at the sides. Inhale, and twist the body in the direction of the bent knee, so that the hands can be placed flat on the floor at the side (see illustration). Exhale and return to starting position. Then change legs and repeat on the other side.

Spinal Twist (*Plate 27*)

Benefits: Stimulates the whole system through its action on the adrenal glands. Increases vitality; invigorates spinal nerves,

massages abdominal organs, exercises the spine, corrects constipation and indigestion; reduces hips, stomach and waistline.

This is a beautiful *asana* and worth doing well, though it is a
little difficult to learn. You could get into it either from Sideways Swing Position or from Cross-Legged Pose.

With the legs crossed, press your left knee down to the floor
and hold it there while you step over it with the right leg. Keep
the right thigh close to the body, with thigh and calf forming a
triangle with the floor. Bend the right arm behind the back.
Stretch out the left arm, and keeping it straight, move it over
the right knee until that knee is under the left armpit, and the
arm (left) lies parallel with and against the right calf. With the
left hand take hold of the right foot. (Consult the illustration.)
Inhale; exhale and slowly twist the body from the waistline, as
far as possible to the right, trying to see behind you. Then come
forward, change sides and repeat.

Sideways Swing (Plate 28)
Benefits: Keeps spine supple. Reduces waistline and hips.

Sit with both legs bent to the left of the body, as in illustration.
Loosely link the arms over the head. Inhale, and as you exhale
swing the body and arms over the bent legs. Swing several times
on one side, then change the legs to other side and repeat.

Pose of a Fish (Plate 29)
Benefits: Facilitates complete yoga abdominal breathing. Corrects constipation. Stimulates ovaries and corrects menstrual
troubles. Keeps spine and hips supple.

The Fish Pose, correctly performed, requires the legs to be
locked in the Lotus Position (see Appendix), but simple cross-
legged pose may be substituted.

Modification of Fish Pose
Cross the legs, lie back on the floor and cross your arms behind
your neck. The right hand is on the left shoulder-blade and the
left hand on the right shoulder-blade, with the head resting on
the crossed arms.

Cobra (Plate 30)
Benefits: Keeps spine supple; stimulates adrenal glands, sex
glands, abdominal organs. Improves constipation and menstrual
troubles.

Lie down on your stomach and put your palms flat on the

floor, about level with your chest. Inhale, raising head, neck and top part of the trunk, putting pressure on the small of the back and keeping the rest of the body pressed to the floor. The spine must be arched backwards with the face looking up. Hold for 5–7 seconds, then come down, exhaling. *The lower part of the body, from the waist down, must be kept pressed to the floor, otherwise there will not be the right pressure on the back and effect of the asana will be lost.*

Practise *Cobra* twice in this way, then twice more, pressing the chin to the chest as you rise up, stimulating the thyroid gland.

Locust (*Plate* 31)

Benefits: Keeps spine supple; improves respiratory system; strengthens abdominal and back muscles and tones up ovaries.

A modified version of this *asana* may be practised by those who cannot manage the full pose.

Lie down on the stomach and bring the arms under the thighs, keeping the elbows straight and the fists clenched. Turn the hands so that the thumbs are underneath. Turn the face to one side. Inhale, and quickly raise both legs into the air, trying to keep them together and straight, and keeping the face on the floor. Exhale and come down.

In the modified version, inhale and raise one leg. Lower it as you exhale. Repeat with the other leg.

Pose of a Camel (*Plate* 32)

Benefits: Keeps the spine supple; tones up spinal nerves, and reproductive organs in women. Firms neck and slims stomach and waistline.

On your knees, with legs slightly apart, arch the back, stretching the arms behind you and resting the hands on the heels. Keep the elbows straight, let the head fall back. Retain position, inhaling and exhaling.

For those whose spines are not very supple it will be necessary to lean back in order to put the hands on the heels, but try to get as much of an arch as possible in the spine.

Pose of a Cat (*Plates* 33 *and* 34)

Benefits: Exercises the spine and keeps it supple. Tones up women's reproductive organs.

On your knees, lean forward and put the palms flat on the floor. Let the head hang down and keep the arms straight. (The arms, trunk and thighs form a rectangle with the floor.) Manipulate your spine, raising and lowering the middle part just like a cat, bringing it up into a hump, then coming down, arching the back, but keeping the arms rigid. All the movement is done with the spine.

Knees-to-Stomach (Plate 35)
Benefits: Stimulates facial tissues. Corrects indigestion and flatulence.

Lie on your back. Inhale and draw the knees up to the stomach, pressing them against the body with the hands and holding them there, with breath retained, until a pressure is felt in the face and head. Then release legs and lower them while exhaling. Repeat several times. (Forbidden in cases of hypertension.)

Headstand (Fig. B)
Benefits: The king of all yoga positions. Rejuvenates the whole body; increases vitality and sex powers; tones up glands, nervous centres and brain. Improves memory, concentration, sinus complaints, asthma, some heart conditions. Benefits eyes, teeth, hair, ears, facial tissues, throat, Correct displaced organs, varicose veins, prolapses and all conditions caused by pull of gravity.

Prohibited for students with high blood pressure, weak eye capillaries, inflammation of ears. If over fifty and very much overweight, to be used with caution. The best rule is to get your doctor's approval.

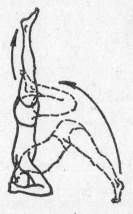

FIG B

123

Kneel down. Lace your fingers together, lean forward and rest forearms and hands on the floor, with the palms facing towards you. Your hands and arms should form a little enclosure. Put your head on the *floor* inside this enclosure, NOT on your hands. The correct spot on the head varies with individuals but generally speaking is between the crown of the head and the hair-line. If too close to the forehead the neck will be bent back; if too far to the back of the head you will overbalance. Experiment till you find the right place.

From this kneeling position, with the head on the floor, straighten out your legs and begin to walk in towards your body. (This is to bring the buttocks up. The body and legs form a triangle with the floor at this stage.) When you feel you are close enough, try to raise your feet from the floor, with the knees bent, gradually lifting and straightening them until the whole body is in one straight line. The back must not be arched and the elbows must be kept fairly close together. Inhale and exhale deeply while holding the pose.

To come down, slowly bring the knees down and in to the stomach, folding yourself up, until the feet touch the floor.

In the beginning you may have to kick yourself up, but as the back muscles become stronger you will lift the legs more slowly. Never practise alone unless against a wall, for you could kick right over your head and fall. Be sure to inhale and exhale while holding the pose, to supply extra oxygen to the blood that is going to the head. Do not hold the Headstand for more than a few seconds in the beginning. Do not practise it after eating or drinking. Do not be persuaded to demonstrate it at parties.

Abdominal contractions: digestive cycle
Benefits: Provides deep internal massage. Cures constipation and indigestion. Tones up all abdominal organs, including reproductive system. Firms stomach. Leads to inner cleanliness.

These *asanas* are considered the most important in yoga, after the Headstand and Candle. They should be learnt and practised by everyone who seeks relief from constipation or who is suffering from sexual debility or menstrual irregularity.

They must not be practised on a full stomach, or for at least three hours after a meal; nor during pregnancy, during menstruation, nor when there are ulcers.

Uddiyana (Plate 36)
Stand with the feet apart, slightly bend the knees and place

your palms on the thighs, rather high up, with the fingers turned inward.* Lean forward with the weight on the heels of the hands, letting the front of the body relax and slightly arching the back. Inhale, completely exhale; then contract the abdominal muscles, drawing the stomach right in and back as though trying to bring it against the spine. The contraction is a slightly upward diagonal movement, for the diaphragm is also raised in the process. The chin is locked to the chest. Hold the contraction, then relax. Inhale, exhale and repeat. (All air must be expelled from the lungs before the contraction.)

When you have mastered this part, try to learn to contract and relax quickly, making a flapping movement in and out several times, before relaxing and taking the next inhalation.

Uddiyana and *Nauli* (see Appendix) are also practised in sitting pose, Crosslegged, Lotus, or Pose of an Adept. The hands rest on the knees, with the fingers turned inward and the weight on the heels of the hands, as above. The same procedure is followed.

Digestive cycle
Sit with the legs crossed and hands resting on the knees. Lean forward from the waist and move the body round in a circular direction to the left, four times; then stop and reverse the movement, circling to the right four times. As you lean forward, push the stomach out; as you lean back, draw it in. The object of the exercise is to massage the abdominal organs and increase the gastric fire.

*See the illustration for *Nauli*, in the Appendix.

11

FACE, NECK, EYES, TEETH, EARS, HAIR

In Chapter 5 we have discussed the general care of the skin, eyes, teeth and ears. In this chapter, specific techniques are suggested which will help to delay, even eradicate, signs of wear and tear in these parts of the body.

Eyes

The yoga eye exercises are part of traditional training to maintain good sight. It is not suggested that they will cure diseases of the eyes or restore poor vision in every case, but failing sight could frequently be arrested and vision improved considerably, if taken in time.

The exercises are usually practised about half-way through a lesson, after the inverted poses, and preceding the forward-stretching cycle. They should be done sitting cross-legged, with the hands resting comfortably on the knees, and back and neck in one straight line.

Only the eyes are moved, and they should be focused each time upon some specific point rather than vaguely directed towards it. This will help to strengthen the power of focusing.

Eye Exercises
Moving only the eyes, and each time focusing upon something:

1. Eyes up, down; up, down; up, down; close.

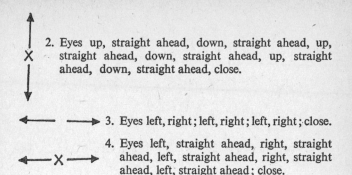

2. Eyes up, straight ahead, down, straight ahead, up, straight ahead, down, straight ahead, up, straight ahead, down, straight ahead, close.

3. Eyes left, right; left, right; left, right; close.

4. Eyes left, straight ahead, right, straight ahead, left, straight ahead, right, straight ahead, left, straight ahead; close.

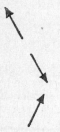

5. Eyes looking up in diagonal direction; then down; up, rightcorner; down, left corner; up, right corner; down, left corner; close.

6. Change; up, left corner; down, right corner, etc.; close.

7. Slowly circling the eyes, right round to the right; close. Slowly circling the eyes, right round to the left; close.

Changing of focus
8. Look at the tip of your nose, then at a point in the distance; nose, distance; nose, distance; close.
9. Look at the tip of your finger, held about a foot away, then distance; finger, distance; finger, distance; close.
10. Practise looking at an object without blinking – not staring in the sense of straining but trying to see it more clearly.
11. Massage the eyes by squeezing the lids tightly together, then blinking rapidly several times.

There are a number of traditional passes which are done at the end of the cycle, using the *prana* or life-force in the fingers.

1. With thumb and forefinger held together, gently stroke the closed eyelids, drawing thumb and finger across from the inner to the outer corner of the eye.
2. Place the palms over the eyes with the fingers closed and resting on the forehead. Gently bring the palms down over the closed eyes in a massaging movement, repeating several times.

   Close the eyes and place the finger-tips gently round the eyeballs (right hand on right eye, left on left) and hold them there, breathing *prana* or life force into the eyes. Since *prana* is said to escape from the body through the finger-tips, this pose directs it to the eyes with strengthening effects.

   Now practise palming, placing the palms of the hands over the eyes to completely exclude the light.

This cycle of exercises could be followed by Sunning the Eyes in appropriate weather, as described on page 59, Chapter 5.

The inverted positions and those that bring blood to the head ... raised poses, swinging down from the waist ... all contribute to healthy eyes by increasing the circulation to the optic nerves; but such exercises should *not* be practised in cases of inflammation, acute irritation, or weak eye capillaries.

Neck exercises

Sitting in the cross-legged position and moving only the head and neck:

1. Lift up the head and then lower it.
2. Turn the head from right to left, from left to right.
3. Slant the head towards one shoulder, then to the other.
4. Lift the head, then let it fall forward, completely relaxing neck muscles.
5. Thrust the chin out, then pull it in. (This is for double-chin.)
6. Circle the head right round to the right; then to the left.
7. Clasp your hands at the back of the neck and push the head down and forward, at the same time resisting with the neck.

This strengthens the muscles at the back of the neck and is an important exercise in preventing Dowager's Hump.

Finish by briskly tapping the back of the neck, the cheeks and under the chin with the finger-tips.

Each movement should be practised at least four times.

You will also help to improve your neck by the following *asanas*: Pose of a Camel (page 122); Cobra (page 121); Supine Pelvic (Appendix, page 150); Spinal Twist (page 120); Bow (Appendix); Fish Pose (page 121); Half-Shoulderstand (page 111); and Headstand (page 123).

Teeth

Apart from the care and attention recommended for the teeth in Chapter 6, their general health will be improved by the following:

Any position in which the chin is locked to the chest . . . Shoulderstand (page 110); Pose of Tranquillity (page 111); and Headstand (page 123); Facial exercises Numbers 4 and 7 on pages 130–1. All other inverted poses and the swinging-down movements on page 93 (limbering-up cycle). The Stretching cycle (pages 118–19); Raised Poses, if possible (see Appendix); *Yoga-mudra* (page 115); Head of a Cow (page 116); Pose of a Hare (page 114); Pose of a Child (page 114).

Ears (see also Chapter 5)

When the circulation slows down, the auditory nerve may be affected by lack of arterial blood.

All the inverted poses . . . Headstand (page 123); and Shoulderstands (page 110) are recommended. All *asanas* that bring blood to the face and head . . . the forward stretching cycle (page 118); Head of a Cow (page 116); *Yoga-mudra* (page 115); Pose of a Hare (page 114); Pose of a Child (page 114); swinging-down movements (page 93) and neck exercises on pages 128–9 and *Refreshing of perceptionary senses*, described on page 138, Mental techniques.

Hair

It has been said that the Headstand will cure baldness; in any case, with the Half-Shoulderstand, it will benefit the hair, for both positions send arterial blood to roots and scalp. Hold the poses long enough to give the blood time to reach the top of the head and concentrate the mind upon directing it there. All the *asanas* and movements recommended for teeth and ears should be practised, and the general care of the hair noted, as described in Chapter 5, page 60.

The scalp should be kept movable, to ensure proper circulation of blood to the roots of the hair. To develop and retain this flexibility, practise moving the scalp back and forth, wrinkling the forehead if necessary to facilitate the action; then massage briskly with the tips of the fingers until a pleasant warmth is felt.

Face. Sagging of facial muscles
(See also Chapter 5 – Care of the Skin)

The effects of central gravity on the face and the results of circulatory weakness have already been mentioned.

Apart from the *asanas* which bring blood to the face and help to prevent and destroy wrinkles, there are a number of facial exercises designed to tighten up sagging muscles and strengthen weakened tissues affected by the pull of gravity. Some of these movements are incorporated in modern methods of face-lifting without surgery.

Regular daily practice is essential for success; and the exercises should be done before a mirror, with the mind fully concentrated upon the desired result. You must be convinced that you will succeed, for self-hypnosis is a very important part of these techniques.

Put your hands gently on the cheeks as you practise and learn to identify the muscles involved. This will help you to perform the movements more intelligently.

Whenever the face feels tired, or begins to look drawn you should tone it up with this cycle. Practise each movement until a pleasant tiredness is felt.

1. *To firm the cheeks.* Slightly puff the cheeks, tensing and relaxing the muscles.
2. *For mouth and lips.* Open and close the mouth, pushing the lips forward so that the movement resembles a fish breathing.
3. *For sagging corners of the mouth.* Move the jaw from side to side.
4. *For toning up cheek muscles, chin and roots of teeth.* Clench

130

the fists and place one on top of the other under the chin, thumbs uppermost. Press them up against the chin and at the same time force the jaw down against them.

5. *For the throat and skin under the chin.* Imagine there is a heavy weight on your chin which you must lift. Raise the chin, tensing the muscles underneath it.

6. *To massage tissues inside face and invigorate facial muscles.* Fill your mouth with air, puff out your cheeks and roll the air round inside, forcing it under top lip, bottom lip, up at the sides of the jaws and into the cheeks.

7. Repeat the process, using the tongue instead of air, massaging whole interior of the mouth, lips, gums and teeth.

8. *For facial muscles.* Tense and relax the teeth at the back of the jaws.

9. *For throat, root of tongue and face.* Practise Pose of a Lion (page 114).

10. *To stimulate circulation.* Briskly tap the face and under the chin with the fingers.

The eye exercises given in this chapter may also be included in this cycle since they tone up the muscles round the eye sockets, a very vulnerable part of the face.

Practise also the mental beauty techniques given in Chapter 12, pages 139–43; and the inverted poses . . . especially Half-Shoulderstand (page 111); and Headstand (page 123); the Raised Poses (pages 148–9); and all those given above for teeth, ears and hair, designed to bring arterial blood to the face.

Conclude with a few minutes of rhythmical breathing, trying to relax all tension in the face and releasing the inner light so often obscured by worry or stress (see page 139, Mental Techniques).

Finally, try to cultivate inner tranquillity and a philosophical attitude to life, for good looks can be spoilt by a discontented, disagreeable expression.

12

MENTAL TRAINING

Life is a turbulent, fast-flowing river; the body is the vessel in which we travel. It must be strengthened if we are to complete our journey without foundering or being swept away from our course. This strength comes from physical training; but the serious student knows that mental and spiritual development are equally important, for it is only through them that he can remain in command of his vessel.

The yogi's complete control of mind over body is achieved through constant practice of techniques designed to bring mastery of the entire self; and since yoga is a path of continuous development, the adept is never satisfied.

Mental powers and moral qualities, like the muscles of the body, need exercising. Like muscles, they may be developed and strengthened, and can atrophy and die for want of use.

Traditionally, mental exercises are practised when the "forces of Soul" are in complete balance, and after the body has been prepared by training and cleansing processes which purify the 72,000 *Nadis* or nervous channels and the seven *Chakras* or nervous centres.

For the western student this could be interpreted as choosing a time when not disturbed, harassed or depressed; and after observing a light, but nourishing diet, preferably vegetarian, for at least forty-eight hours.

Mental exercises should not be practised with a full stomach, nor when hungry. The choice of time and place is also important. The best time is mid-morning; and though practice could be done in the open (in a secluded, peaceful place, in the shade of the trees), a small room, practically bare of furniture is even better for helping the complete concentration of thoughts. Since most of the exercises are done sitting cross-legged, the seat should be sufficiently comfortable for even the most prolonged practice.

The traditional seat is described as a grass mat, covered with a piece of felt, and then with an antelope skin, and in hot weather, with linen. In the west, where antelope is scarce, a foam-rubber mat, 6 feet by 3 feet and 1 inch thick is ideal.

The first requirement for practising mental exercises is the ability to sit steadily in one of the four cross-legged positions for a considerable time. For most western students over forty the simple cross-legged pose is best, though they could experiment with the Pose of an Adept or even the Buddha pose (see page 113).

The cross-legged positions, being physically concentrated poses, help mental concentration, and when they are held for any length of time the brain is stimulated, for blood circulation is slowed down in the legs and increased in the upper part of the body. This is especially so with the Lotus Pose.

Your first exercise will be to sit as still as possible, breathing deeply and rhythmically, gradually increasing the time until eventually you can sit for an hour without difficulty.

Though this exercise is simple, it greatly contributes to the power of concentration and is in itself a powerful tranquillizer.

All mental exercises are preceded by the regulation and slowing down of the breath, which quietens the mind and brings increased receptivity and ability to focus the thoughts.

Sitting in a quiet place, with legs crossed, hands folded or resting lightly on the knees, back and neck in one straight line, shut the eyes to exclude distractions and slow down the breath to the rate of six heart-beats to each inhalation, six to each exhalation. If you cannot time it in your mind, put your finger on your pulse and count the beats as you breathe.

Development of Concentration

Whatever you are doing, whether in yoga or your daily life, you cannot succeed without concentration. The Russian scientist, Pavlov, taught that it is one of the most important manifestations of the human mind; that it was this power alone that enabled man to develop from an ape.

It is essential to yoga training, for with breathing and relaxation it forms the basis of all successful practice.

The power of concentration can be developed by exercise. (The word *concentration* is usually employed when the mind is focused upon one point.) Our minds are very poorly disciplined; they cannot stay for long on any one thing, so in the early stages of training they are given objects upon which to fix themselves . . . a tree, a flower, a cloud . . . It is the process of concentration that is important rather than its subject.

You could start by putting an actual article in front of you and trying to concentrate on it for longer and longer periods. Later, proceed to something abstract . . . a single thought or idea.

Do not be discouraged if at first you cannot hold the object in your mind. This is quite usual and will improve with practice; but always remember that everything in yoga must be done with the power of concentration (constructive thought) supporting the physical action, so that improvement of this power will affect every other aspect of your practice.

Creating a mental ashram

The creating of a spiritual *ashram* or hermitage is an important part of mental training.

No matter how comfortable or well-appointed their houses, urban people often long to get away, to change their environment, to live in the forest or by the sea, and despite primitive conditions, the torments of heat or cold, mosquitoes or wild life they usually come back from these escapes feeling recharged and invigorated, mentally relaxed and refreshed.

This is the thought behind the city-dweller's passion for a weekender, even a boat or car in which he can get away from everything.

The ancient yogis were aware of this instinct in the human mind but they taught that instead of seeking external change, we should turn inward, to our inner selves, finding refreshment there.

The mind holds all and everything . . . forests and seas, the most beautiful corners of the earth, the stars, planets and unknown worlds. In the mind we can travel a thousand miles with the speed of a thought.

It is a tradition that in the very beginning of his training a student creates his own private sanctuary where he can go in time of need, leaving behind all and everything. For those who perfect the method these escapes become a real exit from the usual environment, mentally invigorating and refreshing.

The spiritual retreat is usually a garden, "full of tall trees, shrubs, flowers, and meditative shrines", but you could create anything that satisfies your own personality . . . an island, a remote monastery, a hidden valley in the Himalayas . . . You should not describe it to anyone. Keep it entirely for yourself. Whenever you need mental rest it is there ready for you.

When you enter this *ashram* in the last stage of *Savasana* (Pose of complete rest) you complete your relaxation in a different world.

Concentration on breath

Under normal conditions and in good health we are not conscious of breathing, but when the mind is concentrated on the process of inhalation and exhalation a strange phenomenon is experienced, even by a new student.

Through concentration on breath you become detached from your physical body, quickly losing all consciousness of its existence, feeling light and free as a breath. This is the purpose of the exercise, and leads to complete relaxation of the nerves. It is a powerful tranquillizer and a natural tonic for the entire nervous system. In healing yoga it is used to cure a host of such minor maladies as headaches, toothache and so on.

Creating of a flower

This may also be done either in *Savasana* or one of the cross-legged positions.

Concentrate on evoking the image of a familiar flower, using your Mind's Eye, and trying to see it in every detail. You must *see* it, not just think about it; and the image must be held steadily while you examine its shape, colour, texture, formation. Then try to smell its scent as you inhale.

The exercise develops the power of imagination and brings complete mental relaxation.

Conversation with the Vital Organs

With pose and breath established, concentrate your mind in turn on the different organs of the body . . . the heart, stomach, kidneys, liver, etc. . . . . with every exhalation sending *prana*, goodwill, and encouragement.

In your mind you actually *talk* to your vital organs; and yoga teaches that if the right amount of concentration is produced the organs will listen attentively and obey the commands of the Master Mind.

Protective Cocoon

As you exhale, direct *prana* through all the hair-pores of the skin (see page 85, Breathing) with the mind concentrated upon the image of an invisible envelope or cocoon forming round your body, shutting you in from external distractions, worries, interruptions, even from heat and cold. With the necessary concentration this exercise becomes a powerful method of refreshing the mind and body, an escape from all and everything that normally harasses and disturbs.

Goodwill breath of the Yogi

This important exercise is based on the yoga belief that every cell in the body possesses its own instinctive mind and that by persistent training one could achieve direct control of them.

Establish steady pose and steady breath. Close your eyes and visualize your body as millions of living cells. Imagine that you are in direct communication with the instinctive minds ruling the lives of the cells, and with each exhalation send a goodwill message, and a stream of *prana* or life force to each one.

In the higher stages of training, an adept can attain remarkable powers of self-healing through this exercise. There are many recorded examples of the fully-trained yogi's ability to speed up the natural healing processes tenfold.

Blankness of the Mind

Blankness is the ability to wipe out all thoughts, and impulses of thoughts from the mind, trying to attain the condition experienced while unconscious or in a deep sleep. You must not fall asleep in this exercise but for a few minutes try to make your mind really blank. Technically it is easier to achieve by looking up with the eyes closed.

Idleness of Mind

Idleness of mind is a state of pleasant nothingness that is restful and refreshing. A sage of the past, describing this exercise, compared the mind to a blue sky, and the thoughts to lazily-rolling clouds.

It is usually practised in *Savasana* (lying flat on the back, completely relaxed). Try to withdraw every bit of tension, conscious and sub-conscious, from your mind, and give yourself over to the feeling that nothing matters.

Floating on a Cloud

This exercise, as practised by ancient sages, is said to develop powers of levitation, but for modern students its main value is in its soothing effect on the nervous system.

It may be done sitting cross-legged or lying on the back. Concentrate on the thought that with each exhalation you are sending a stream of *prana* against the forces of gravity; that with each outgoing breath your body is growing lighter and lighter. After some time of concentration there is an actual sensation of extreme lightness, and a pleasant feeling of floating in the air, brought about by complete relaxation of the nerves.

Development of the Mind's Eye

The Mind's Eye (also known as the Third Eye) is one of the most extraordinary faculties of the human mind. Apart from the ability to see into the past, to re-create an object hundreds of miles away or the face of a friend long dead, it is the power to see what the physical eyes can never see at all.

A yogi can train himself to see into his own body, achieving greater mastery over it through increased knowledge of its functioning.

Development of the Mind's Eye is an important part of training for it is used in many physical exercises, as, for example, in the second part of *Savasana* when it is turned in on the self . . . trying to *see* the pockets of inner tension and so relax them completely. It is also used in many *asanas*, movements and gestures, when the student learns to *see* the movements of joints, vertebrae, glands, or vital organs.

The exercise should be done regularly and methodically, at the same time every day.

Sit down in one of the cross-legged positions, establish deep and rhythmical breathing, close your eyes and concentrate on the point between the eyebrows . . . seat of the Third Eye. Try to see clearly and *in colour*, a tree that you know, or perhaps your dinner table the night before, in full detail. You may use all sorts of objects, landscapes, faces, concentrating on developing the ability to actually *see* them as clearly as you can.

If you are one of the people who can only see in black and white, learn to see in colour, as vividly as possible. You might even get a paintbox and actually mix the colours that you see with your Mind's Eye, then compare them with those of the real objects.

This is a fascinating exercise and excellent training for artists and writers or anyone to whom a well-developed Mind's Eye is important.

Stillness of the Mind

Stillness of the mind is a highly esteemed yogic practice which is a necessary preliminary to meditation, and is in itself an experience on an entirely different plane of consciousness.

"In complete stillness of body and mind a light is born," Master Lu-Tzu taught, suggesting that dimensional, earth-bound thoughts obscure the higher vision. "Life holds no secrets for the yogi who is capable of stilling his mind at will". Knowledge through esoteric experience could be attained by this exercise.

Because it involves disciplining our unruly minds it is a most difficult exercise and requires great persistence. Sit in a cross-legged position, with deep and rhythmical breath established, and try to gradually eliminate all thoughts *while still keeping the mind alert and receptive to higher vibrations*.

In this exercise the mind might be compared to a balloon and the thoughts to the strings holding it to the ground. When the strings are cut, the mind, like a balloon, soars high up into a different plane of consciousness.

Face Gesture

This is a strange and often misinterpreted yoga method. Its aim is to invigorate the perceptionary senses through conscious effort.

It is practised in the cross-legged position.

Exhale completely, then close the ears, eyes, nostrils and mouth, using thumbs, index fingers, middle and fourth fingers respectively.

Retain the pose for about ten seconds.

It is said that through practising Face Gesture, one improves the senses of hearing, seeing, smelling, tasting and touching.

Mirror of the Mind

Sit cross-legged with eyes closed and establish breathing. Concentrate on evoking the image of yourself, as though you were looking into a mirror. Persevere until you can hold the image steadily in your mind; then project it into the future, unchangeable. The thought behind your concentration is of the years ahead, the passage of time, and yourself still looking as you do now. You see, and hold the image of yourself, unchanged and never changing.

In a further stage of the exercise, having created the present image, you then evoke yourself as you were twenty years ago – whatever period you like – and try to fit this younger image over the present one, completely obscuring it.

This technique is a form of dual self-hypnosis in which you actually hypnotize your mind, using your own mind as the instrument.

Intense concentration is said to result in a rejuvenated appearance.

Releasing of Inner Light

This technique is quite different from *Concentration on Inner Light* (page 146), although it is directly connected with the light within us.

We are hiding our inner light behind a façade of tension. If we can learn to release this tension the light will shine through, illuminating and beautifying the features. (People usually look younger and more handsome in sleep – and sometimes just after death – because all tension is relaxed.)

Sit down with the legs crossed, establish deep breathing and concentrate on relaxing every bit of tension in your face. More and more inner light will shine through as you relax. There is no limit to this technique of enlightenment.

This physical-spiritual exercise is an important part of *avatara* yoga, and is used for graceful ageing. Only a completely developed *avatara* is capable of total arresting of the ageing process. (There have been very few *avataras* in the whole history of the human race. See note on page 18.)

Inversion of the Mind's Eye

In this exercise the Mind's Eye is turned in, not upon your physical body but your inner self. You are making an honest attempt to know yourself, to face up to your faults and weaknesses, without evasion or excuse.

Use this self-analysis constructively, in further exercises such as:

Development of Inner Strength

With the mind withdrawn from external influences, concentrate on the thought of developing Inner Strength. Resolve that you *will* be strong in the face of temptation, hardship, trial. That you will not take the easy way out, that you can hold on, however difficult or frustrating your life may seem, and that it is only you who can help yourself.

This exercise is practised either in Cross-legged Pose, or in Pose of a Hero, which is said to develop inner strength.

Development of Will-power

Concentrate on the thought that if mental and moral powers are not used they will atrophy, like muscles; that you will not let your will-power fade, that you will exercise it constructively at every opportunity. As a beginning you could make up your mind to do some disagreeable task that you have been avoiding for some time. Resolve that you will keep on trying to improve until you are able to face even the most difficult moral situations with courage and serenity.

The Seven Fears

The seven fears are connected with possessions, friends, health, loneliness, love, death and fear itself.

A real yogi must learn to overcome all these fears and completely liberate his mind from their destructive influence.

To practise the exercise, take each fear in turn and try to develop a constructive attitude towards it. Instead of brooding on deprivation, concentrate on what may be salvaged from the wreck (which may never happen), on what the experience could teach you, on the wisdom and spiritual strength that is often the outcome of severe trials.

The following themes are suggested for meditation on the individual fears –

1. Fear of losing possessions
Concentrate on the thought of the ephemeral value of all material possessions and on the everlasting value of an awakened spirit.

2. Loss of friends
Concentrate on the thought that true friendship cannot be destroyed by physical separation.

3. Loss of health
A true yogi does his best to maintain good health, but if illness comes, accepts it philosophically as a manifestation of *karma*,* while doing what he can to combat it.

4. Fear of loneliness
The yogi knows that when he is alone he is with God Himself. This thought banishes all fear of loneliness.

5. Loss of love
Love is the strongest power in the universe. It is the true light; it is God; it cannot be destroyed. Concentration on this thought conquers fear of losing love.

6. Fear of death
The second part of every thinking person's life should be a preparation for death, in the spiritual sense.

Yoga philosophy does not believe in death as a complete extermination of the individual. It teaches that the soul is immortal. We are all passing through cycles of incarnations, and the yogi's whole life is an attempt to prepare for those incarnations, to achieve a further stage of development.

The acceptance of this belief gives complete freedom from fear of death and brings a noble serenity in the face of the final liberation of the spirit.

Karma. See page 73.

7. *Fear of fear*

Shut your eyes and concentrate on the thought "*I am stronger than fear*". Think of fear as a weakness and determine to overcome it. Think of it as a form of slavery and resolve to free yourself. Think of it as degrading and humiliating and decide that you will regain your dignity and pride. List all your fears, mental and physical, and analyse each one constructively, trying to see what you can do to eradicate it; and form the habit of thinking "in opposites" . . . whenever the thought of fear – in the abstract – comes to your mind, replace it with the thought of courage. Do this not only while sitting cross-legged at your exercises but during your daily life. Use the power of auto-suggestion to train yourself into freedom and strength. Try to believe that *All experience is an arch wherethro' Gleams that untravelled world, whose margin fades Forever and for ever when I move.*

I am Master of Myself

Now you are concentrating on overcoming the weaknesses uncovered in Inversion of the Mind's Eye. All the things you dislike in yourself, all such negative qualities as laziness, greed, envy, possessiveness, procrastination, untruthfulness, hypocrisy, self-indulgence must be taken, one at a time, and weeded out. Concentrate on the opposite of each weakness, the positive quality with which you would like to replace it . . . generosity, self-control, honesty and so on, no matter how long it takes.

Sorting the Seeds of Thought

This exercise is designed to develop positive, constructive thinking and banish negative thoughts.

Impulse is the origin of thought. Yoga calls it the "seed" of thought, and our minds are full of these seeds, both positive and negative.

Sitting in complete stillness of body, with breath established, learn how to sort the seeds, fertilizing the positive and destroying the negative, analysing yourself in deep meditation.

The exercise should be practised regularly. You should return to it again and again, like "a wise gardener returning to his garden daily, watering plants and flowers and destroying weeds".

For a *Karma yogi* (one who chooses the path of action), this exercise is very important in helping him achieve success in life.

Concentration on the object of love and devotion

It does not matter who or what you choose to concentrate upon in this exercise . . . whether it is a person, a place, a spiritual experience . . . it is the force of love evoked that is important.

Holding the object of your greatest love and devotion in your mind, concentrate all your thoughts upon it, letting the warm and life-giving force of love completely fill your being.

Attunement to universal goodness

Concentrate on the thought of all the goodness in the world; that the universe is filled with this quality; on all the unselfishness, helpfulness, nobility, kindness that surround you; on the thought that God is good. Try to identify yourself with this stream of bliss, dissolving the bonds of your own personality and becoming one with it.

Chakra breathing

In the higher stages of yoga training the student encounters a very involved and complex theory about the *chakras* or nervous plexuses (see Chapter 7).

The seven *chakras* or nervous centres of the physical-subtle body mentioned in the traditional yoga scripts are: *Muladara; Svadistana; Manipura; Anahata; Vishuddha; Agna;* and *Brahma*. They are set in the base of the spine, the genitals, the solar plexus, the middle of the chest (vagus nerve), region of the thyroid gland, the point between the eyebrows (the Third Eye) and the top of the head. These *chakras* are credited with physical and occult powers, but all methods of interfering with them – except the three given here – are considered very dangerous and should not be practised without personal guidance.

The following exercises may be performed quite safely.

Sit in one of the cross-legged poses, with eyes shut, hands resting on the knees and establish deep and rhythmical breathing.

Concentrate alternatively on each of the seven *chakras*, starting from the base of the spine, and sending *prana* or life force to each one with every exhalation. Try actually to imagine a stream of *prana*, golden in colour, directed to each of these centres. Learn their positions by heart so that your concentration is not interrupted.

Also concentrate upon the qualities associated with each *chakra*, taking them in the same order from the base of the spine upwards . . . physical purity; control of sex; accumulation of vital force; defying time (ageing); perfection of metabolical processes; spiritual enlightenment; and unity with God.

Only three breaths are allowed to each *chakra* (twenty-one breaths in all), and the rate of breathing must be extremely slow.

Concentration on Manipura chakra, or solar plexus

Concentration on this *chakra*, while breathing, is frequently performed in hatha yoga.

It is done either sitting cross-legged or lying flat on the back. With each exhalation direct *prana* to the solar plexus, concentrating on the thought that the amount of life-force is increased with each inhalation-exhalation.

The finger-tips may be placed on the region of the plexus, the mind visualizing the *prana* streaming from them into the *chakra*. The exercise may be practised as long as you like, and there is no limit to the number of breaths.

Concentration on the Third Eye (Agna chakra)

In this exercise the breath is directed to the point between the eyebrows. The student forms an image of *prana* entering this centre, with revitalizing effects, leading, in this case, to spiritual enlightenment. It brings a sensation of great peace, bliss, perfect balance and happiness, and is often practised before meditation.

The modern leucotomy, the operation which is said to favourably change a patient's personality, even removing criminal tendencies, is performed in the area of the *agna chakra*. Once more it would appear that science and ancient yoga are in agreement, though the surgeon uses a knife and the yogi uses breath and the power of his mind.

Astral Breath

Although the existence of the astral or subtle body has not been proved by science, the rites of certain churches (including Greek and Russian Orthodox) suggest a belief similar to the yogic teaching on this subject.

According to yoga, the astral body is a non-material replica of the human body, dwelling within its physical twin. It has an important influence on physical and mental health, and after death survives the gross body by forty days.

As though recognizing this, both Greek and Russian churches hold a second service on the fortieth day after a death, repeating some of the prayers said at the first service (at the time of the death).

In the *Astral Breath of a Yogi*, breathing cycles are repeated in which one breath is dedicated to the physical body and the second to the astral body. It is practised either in cross-legged position or in *Savasana*, lying completely relaxed on the back. With the breaths the mind should be concentrated alternatively on physical and astral bodies.

Concentration on Inner Sound

"What do you like best in your practice, oh enlightened one?" a *chela* asked his *guru*.

"To sit in complete stillness of body and mind and listen to the music of my soul".

Pythagoras said that the music of the soul was the music of the spheres. Yoga says that it is the beginning of all the music in the world. It is always present within us, but distracted by external sounds, we cannot hear it.

If we learn how to detach ourselves from these external sounds, now to turn the "mind's ear" inward we will hear it again, enlightening the mind and pacifying the spirit.

Sit in the cross-legged position and establish breath; then make an effort to detach yourself from the actual sense of hearing.

145

With increasing concentration, external sounds become muffled and then start to exist *independently*. (Yoga teaches that at this stage a protective aura has been formed round the student); and after further concentration, an inner sound, the "music of the soul" will be heard.

This is not an easy exercise and is not likely to be achieved at the first attempt. It requires highly developed concentration, mental readiness (an open mind) and consistent practice.

Concentration on Inner Light

Concentration on Inner Light is even more advanced than on "Inner Sound".

Inner light is referred to in the ancient scripts as the True Light, the Divine Spark, the Light Of The Spirit, *Atman* (individual soul).

To "see" this light with the Mind's Eye is to realize the truth of reincarnation and the immortality of the soul.

It will be achieved only by a really enlightened student after prolonged meditation, deep and rhythmical breathing, preceded by three days of preparation . . . the first of complete fasting, except for water, the second drinking only fruit juice and the third eating only solid fruit.

Meditation

The true nature of meditation will never be understood by one who is not ready, for above all it demands an open mind and an enlightened soul.

Meditation is self-realization, inspired by a desire for improvement and development; an attempt to sum up one's real spiritual and mental values.

Subjects other than self-realization may also be taken: the immortality of the soul; God; the universe; victory over death, or any similar theme.

In the East, meditation is defined as two stages: Gathering of the Light, which is a preliminary stilling of the mind, and Meditation itself. The traditional position is the cross-legged pose, with steady breath established and the Mind's Eye turned inward. The perceptionary senses are deliberately dulled, or turned off completely.

A simple exercise in self-realization which could be practised by any western student is *Meditation on the day to come and the day just passed*.

In the morning, turn your thoughts ahead, using your knowledge of what you expect to do during the day, and resolve that you will try to act well under all circumstances; that you will meet unexpected difficulties with courage, resource and good humour; that you will do your best to be kind, generous, understanding and honest in all your dealings.

In the evening, think back over the day, analysing events and your own behaviour with detachment, honestly admitting mistakes you may have made, or weaknesses or faults you may have shown, and determining that you will correct them.

APPENDIX

The *asanas* described and illustrated in this section have not been included in the main part of the book because they are advanced and rather too strenuous for many people over forty. We have included them to show what can be done by older pupils but do not suggest that everyone should try them.

The ages of the demonstrators are given with the text.

Pose of a Bird (Age 51, plate 37)

Benefits: Preserves or restores relative strength. Rejuvenates through bringing blood to the face and head. Invigorates the whole system. Increases or restores confidence.

Start from a squatting position with the toes together and the knees wide apart. The arms are held between the knees, with the palms on the floor and the fingers spread out like a bird's claws. The inside of the legs should be pressed against the outside of the arms. Inhale and rise up on your toes, leaning forward and *riding* on your arms until you can lift your toes from the floor, as shown in the picture. Hold for a couple of seconds, then come down, exhaling. It is a balancing position and must be done slowly and smoothly. If you try to jump you will not be able to hold it and may overbalance.

Pose of a Raven (Age – over 50, plate 38)

Benefits: As above.

This is a variation of the Bird Pose, in which both arms are on one side of the knees instead of between them. It is done on the right side and then the left.

Right aspect. Squat on the floor with knees and toes together, and with both arms outside the left knee. Inhale, and rise up on the toes, then forward in a diagonal direction, leaning the weight of the knees against the right arm, riding the arm as in Bird Pose. (See picture.) Exhale and come down; then repeat on the other side.

148

Pose of a Peacock (Age 51, plate 39)

Benefits: As well as benefits given above, the Peacock Pose stimulates the liver, abdominal organs and solar plexus, through the pressure of the elbows in that area.

The body is extended, face downwards, with the upper part raised so that the arms can be placed underneath. The toes are pointed but not dug in to the floor. Put the palms flat on the floor, with the fingers turned towards the feet. The elbows are bent and pressed into the abdomen. Inhale and slowly move the body forward over the arms, keeping the legs straight. As the head and shoulders move forward the legs begin to rise from the ground, and all the weight is taken on the wrists and hands. The forearms become the peacock's legs. Hold briefly, then exhale and come down.

This is a strenuous *asana* and requires strong wrists, but the necessary strength may be developed by practice.

Position of Eight Curves (Age 60, plate 40)

Benefits: Maintains lightness; rejuvenates and invigorates; stimulates the nervous centres along the spinal cord. Increases or restores confidence.

Sit down with legs stretched, knees slightly bent and ankles crossed. If the left foot is uppermost, insert the right arm between the thighs, with elbow slightly bent and palm on the floor. The left arm is outside the body in line with the right.

Inhale and raise the body from the floor, in a slightly forward, diagonal movement, with the face and left shoulder moving downward and the hips and legs coming up. (See illustration.) The right leg is locked with the right elbow and the left foot locked with the right foot. The weight is taken on the palms. Hold for about 30 seconds, exhale coming down and repeat on the other side.

Scorpion (Age 58, plate 41)

Benefits: See Headstand.
Come up into the Headstand (page 123). Arch the back and let the legs come down as far as possible towards the head. (In the complete pose they are resting on the head.)

Very carefully separate the hands and spread them apart, raising the head and face as high as possible. (See picture.) The back must be well arched and head and legs adjusted to give perfect balance.

This photograph was taken just before the *asana* was finished, while the hands were in the process of separation. In the final stage they are flat on the floor.

Bound Headstand (Age 48, plate 42)

Benefits: See Headstand.

This can only be practised by those who have no difficulty in locking the legs in the lotus-position.

Come up into the headstand; then carefully bend one leg, trying to bring the foot down towards the groin, into the half-lotus. Then repeat the process with the other leg until both are locked.

In the beginning it is a help to get someone to put the legs into position for you.

Fish Pose (Age 48, plate 43)

Benefits: Enables the lungs to be completely filled and completely emptied of air; is thus an important pose for deep breathing and is said to relieve many respiratory and bronchial conditions. It is recommended that the Fish Pose be performed after the Plough Position (page 119) for it counteracts any strain or stiffness that might be experienced after this *asana*, by bending the spine the opposite way to that carried out in the Plough.

The legs should be locked in the Lotus Position. Lean back, lower the body to the floor, arching the spine and resting on the crown of the head. The arms may either be stretched forward with the hands holding the toes, or they may be folded under the back of the neck. A third position is to stretch them out on the floor above the head.

Supine Pelvic Pose (Age 51, plate 44)

Benefits: Strengthens the spine; firms thighs and neck; corrects constipation, indigestion and sexual debility. Has a beneficial effect on reproductive system in women.

Sit back on the heels, keeping the legs together. Lean back, arching the spine and taking the weight on the elbows, until the crown of the head rests on the floor. Hands are held in position of prayer. Hold the pose, inhaling and exhaling, as long as comfortable.

An alternative version is to split the heels and sit between them with the buttocks on the floor; then lean back as above. This variation does not arch the spine so much, but it requires very supple knee joints.

Noose Pose (Age 48, plate 45)

Benefits: Develops extreme limberness of joints.
Sitting on the floor, raise the right leg and put it over the shoulder with the calf behind the head; then raise the left in the same way and lock the feet as shown in the illustration. The arms are threaded through the locked legs and placed on the floor, palms down.

Nauli (Age over 50, plate 47)

Benefits: Corrects constipation, indigestion, sexual debility, menstrual disorders. Massages entire region of the abdomen.

Inhale, exhale and draw back the stomach as described in *Uddiyana* (page 124). Then try to separate the abdominal recti muscles by making a downward, thrusting contraction at the pit of the stomach. This is the base of these muscles and if you can master the contraction in this area they will automatically respond and form into a hard column up the centre of the abdomen. (See illustration.) Practise until you can effect this separation; then try the same procedure on the right side, then the left of the abdomen, in each case forming a hard ridge, with the rest of the abdomen hollow. When you have finally managed to separate all three sets you can learn to contract them, one after the other in turn, quickly, in a rotating, wave-like movement . . . centre, right, centre, left, centre, right and so on. In appearance it is a continuous movement.

151

Pose of a Bow (Age 48, plate 46)

Benefits: Strengthens and exercises spine. Stimulates adrenal glands. Firms bust, stomach and thighs. Tones up reproductive organs and glands.

Lying on the floor, face downward, take hold of the heels and, inhaling, pull the legs up, at the same time raising head and shoulders. Exhale and come down.

ASANAS AND EXERCISES TO DELAY AGEING AND IMPROVE VARIOUS CONDITIONS

AGEING, TO DELAY
Full practice, mental and physical, with special emphasis on Headstand; Half-shoulderstand; Shoulderstand. All swinging-downward exercises and Slow Movements in Chapter 9; Raised Poses. All breathing cycles; Recharging of Vital Energy; *Uddiyana; Nauli; Savasana; Yoga-mudra. Mental Exercises:* Mind Mirror; Releasing of Inner Light; Concentration on Love and Devotion.

ANKLES, SWOLLEN
Headstand; Inverted Poses; *Vajroli-mudra;* Exercises in Chapter 9.

ARMS, TO FIRM
Arm exercises in Chapter 9. Raised Poses. Head of a Cow Pose.

ARTHRITIS
All *asanas* and exercises possible.

ASTHMA
All abdominal breathing. Pose of a Frog; Pose of a Fish; *Savasana.*

BACKACHE:
FROM DISPLACED ORGANS – Headstand; Inverted Poses; *Aswini mudra.*

FROM WEAK MUSCLES – Back exercises in Chapter 9; Plough;* Cobra.*

FROM MENSTRUATION* – Spinal Twist;* Fish;* Locust;* Camel;* Headstand. Breathing away pain; Sending *prana* to spine.

BUST, TO FIRM
Cobra; Camel; Bust exercises in Chapter 9.

CHIN, TO PREVENT DOUBLE AND FIRM UNDERNEATH
Pose of a Camel; Supine Pelvic; Face exercises in Chapter 11; Pose of a Lion.

CIRCULATORY TROUBLES
Triangular Pose. All exercises in Chapter 9. Inverted Poses. Breathing cycles.

COLDS
    All breathing cycles, specially Blacksmith's Bellows; Head-
    stand; Shoulderstand; Vital Energy charging.

CONCENTRATION, TO IMPROVE
    Headstand; Half-shoulderstand; Lotus Pose; Balancing
    Poses; *Yoga-mudra;* All concentration exercises in Chapter 12.

CONFIDENCE, LOSS OF
    Headstand; Raised Poses; Cobra; Spinal Twist; Lotus
    Pose; Balancing Poses; *Vajroli-mudra;* Angular Pose;
    Mental exercises in Chapter 12.

CONSTIPATION
    Uddiyana; Nauli; Head-to-knee; Plough; Fish; Cobra;
    Savasana; Locust; Inverted Poses; *Yoga-mudra; Aswini-
    mudra; Vajroli-mudra.*

DEPRESSION
    General practice, especially *Savasana;* Headstand and all
    inverted poses; Cobra; *Vajroli-mudra;* Locust; Spinal
    Twist; Breathing cycles; Mental exercises in Chapter 12;
    Read also Chapter 3 – *Diet.*

DOWAGER'S HUMP
    Neck exercises in Chapter 9. Pose of a Camel; Headstand;
    Inverted Poses.

ENERGY, VITAL – LOSS OF
    Headstand; Shoulderstand; *Savasana; Vajroli-mudra;*
    Breathing cycles; Recharging cycles; Energy-charging
    cycles; Circulating Life Force.

FACIAL MUSCLES, SAGGING
    Inverted Poses; Headstand; Facial exercises in Chapter 11.
    Head of a Cow; *Yoga-mudra.*

FEAR
    Pose of a Hero; Lotus Pose; Headstand; Shoulderstand
    Vajroli-mudra; Spinal Twist; Cobra; Meditation; Mental
    exercises, specially on Fear.

FEET, SWOLLEN
    Inverted poses; Feet exercises in Chapter 9. Read Chapter
    3 – Care of the feet.

    COLD
    Circulation Exercises in Chapter 9. Warming breath.
    Triangular Pose.

FLATULENCE
    Knee-to-stomach Pose; Digestive cycles; Breathing cycles.

FRUSTRATION

GENERAL
Breathing cycles; *Savasana;* Lotus Pose; All mental exercises in Chapter 12; Read Chapter 3.

SEXUAL
Dangerous Pose, and transmuting of energies.

HAEMORRHOIDS
Inverted poses; *Aswini-mudra;* walking on buttocks in Chapter 9; Massage on page 34.

HEARING, FAILING
Headstand; Half-shoulderstand; All forward-swinging exercises in Chapter 9; *Yoga-mudra.*

HEART CONDITIONS
Savasana; Breathing cycles for slowing down breath and heart. Mental exercises in Chapter 12; Read Chapter 3; Pose of a Frog; Pose of a Child; Diamond Pose. Lotus Pose; Fish Pose; in some cases, with doctors permission, Headstand.

HOT FLUSHES
Savasana; Shoulderstand; Quiet breathing cycles; Cooling breath.

HYPERTENSION
Savasana; Pacifying breathing cycles; Frog Pose; Cross-legged Poses; Fish Pose; Diamond Pose; Mental exercises in Chapter 12. Read also Chapters 2 and 3.

IMPOTENCE
Headstand; Shoulderstand; *Savasana; Aswini-mudra; Vajroli-mudra;* Breathing cycles; Transmuting of energies; Read Chapter 6.

INDIGESTION
Digestive cycles; Stomach contractions; *Savasana;* Knees-to-stomach; Head-to-knee; Pacifying Breaths; *Vajroli-mudra; Yoga-mudra;* Forward-stretching.

INSOMNIA
Spinal massage – rocking; Triangular Pose; *Savasana;* Breathing cycles; Plough; Locust; Head-to-knee; Read Chapter 5.

JOINTS, STIFFNESS OF
All general practice, with emphasis on all exercises in Chapter 9; Lotus Pose; Forward-stretching cycle; Spinal Twist; Archer; Camel; Eagle; Fish.

LEGS, TO IMPROVE AND FIRM
Eagle; Angular Pose; Forward-stretching cycle; Lotus;

Head-to-knee; Exercises in Chapter 9.

MEMORY, FAILING

Headstand; *Yoga-mudra;* Pose of a Hare; Exercises bringing blood to the head. Mental exercises in Chapter 12.

MENOPAUSE

Savasana; Breathing and recharging cycles; Cobra; Spinal Twist; Head-to-knee; Stomach contractions; *Aswini-mudra;* Shoulderstand; Mental exercises in Chapter 12; Read Chapter 6.

MENSTRUAL DIFFICULTIES

Shoulderstand; Plough; Fish; Locust; Stomach contractions; *Aswini-mudra;* Cobra; Head-to-knee; *Savasana.*

MIGRAINE

Savasana; Headstand; Breathing cycles.

NECK, TO FIRM

Neck exercises in Chapter 11; Pose of a Camel.

PROLAPSE

Headstand and all inverted poses; *Aswini-mudra;* Abdominal contractions (with doctor's approval).

PROSTATE GLAND, ENLARGEMENT

Aswini-mudra; Arch gesture.

RELATIVE STRENGTH, LOSS OF

Raised poses (Appendix).

RHEUMATISM

Spinal Twist; Cobra; Locust and general practice.

SCIATICA

Spinal Twist.

SEXUAL DEBILITY

Headstand; Shoulderstand; *Vajroli-mudra;* Half-shoulderstand; Plough; Fish; Eagle; *Aswini-mudra;* Frog Pose; Spinal Twist; *Uddiyana.* Transmutation of energies.

SIGHT, CARE OF

Eye exercises in Chapter 11; Read also Chapter 5. Headstand; Half-shoulderstand; *Yoga-mudra;* All forward-swinging exercises.

SINUS TROUBLE

Headstand; Breathing cycles; Blacksmith's Bellows.

STOMACH, TO FIRM AND SLIM

Uddiyana; Nauli; Camel; Locust; Forward-stretching cycle; Archer; Spinal Twist; *Vajroli-mudra;* All stomach exercises in Chapter 9.

STRESS AND TENSION

Savasana; Shoulderstand; Pacifying breaths; Balancing

Poses; Angular Pose; Cross-legged Poses; Diamond Pose; Pose of a Frog; Read Chapter 2. Mental exercises in Chapter 12.

TEETH

Headstand; Half-shoulderstand; Face and neck exercises; Read Chapters 5 and 11.

THIGHS, TO FIRM

Exercises in Chapter 9; Cobra; Locust; Lotus; Star Pose; Head-to-knee; Supine pelvic (Appendix).

THROAT, WEAKNESS OF

Pose of a Lion; Breathing cycles; Shoulderstand.

THYROID DEFICIENCY

Shoulderstand; Cobra with chin pressed in; Choking Pose; Recharging breaths; Mental exercises.

ULCERS

Savasana; Breathing cycles; Fish Pose; Pose of a Frog; Diamond Pose; Read Chapters 2 and 3; All mental exercises in Chapter 12.

VARICOSE VEINS

All inverted poses, including Headstand. Read also page 33, Chapter 2.

WAISTLINE, TO REDUCE

Sideways swing; Exercises in Chapter 9. Spinal Twist; Cobra; Forward-stretching cycle.

WEIGHT

EXCESS

Shoulderstand; All general practice. Read Chapters 2 and 4 – *Diet*.

DEFICIENCY

Shoulderstand; *Savasana;* Breathing cycles; Exercises in Chapter 9; Read Chapter 4 – *Diet*.

WORRY

All breathing cycles; Recharging with energy; Shoulderstand; *Savasana;* Pose of a Hero; Pose of a Frog; Fish Pose; Lotus Pose; Mental exercises in Chapter 12; Read Chapters 2 and 3.

WRINKLES

Headstand; Half-shoulderstand; Knee-to-stomach; Face exercises in Chapter 11; *Yoga-mudra;* All forward-stretching movements; Pose of a Camel. Head of a Cow.

PROHIBITIONS

Blood-pressure – hypertension: No inverted poses; no breathing exercises that increase pressure in the head; no swinging down

157

from the waist; nothing that brings blood to the head.

Weak eye capillaries: As above.

Inflamed ears or eyes: As above.

Varicose veins: No positions that slow down circulation in legs . . . e.g. Lotus, sitting back on heels, Supine pelvic . . . or put pressure on leg veins.

Prolapse of uterus: No strenuous raised poses.

Stomach contractions

Not to be practised until three hours after meals; not to be done during menstruation or pregnancy or in the case of ulcers.

Sphere books include:

ISOMETRIC WAY TO INSTANT FITNESS	W. H. Rankin	4/-
PEARS MEDICAL ENCYCLOPAEDIA	J. A. C. Brown	7/6
GREAT DISHES OF THE WORLD	Robert Carrier	10/6
THE FACE OF WAR	Martha Gellhorn	5/-
YOGA OVER FORTY	Michael Volin Nancy Phelan	5/-
ULYSSES FOUND	Ernle Bradford	4/6
FAR BOUNDARIES	August Derleth	3/6
A STANDARD OF BEHAVIOUR	William Trevor	3/6
THE SECOND OSWALD	Richard H. Popkin	4/6
A SILVER PLATED SPOON	Duke of Bedford	5/-
SHORT HISTORY OF RUSSIAN REVOLUTION	Joel Carmichael	5/-
HERE COMES THE TOFF	John Creasey	3/6
THE TOFF GOES TO MARKET	John Creasey	3/6
THE TOFF PROCEEDS	John Creasey	3/6
DOUBLE FOR THE TOFF	John Creasey	3/6
THE D.A. CALLS A TURN	Erle Stanley Gardner	2/6
THE D.A. COOKS A GOOSE	Erle Stanley Gardner	2/6
THE D.A. GOES TO TRIAL	Erle Stanley Gardner	2/6
CLUE OF THE FORGOTTEN MURDER	Erle Stanley Gardner	2/6
CASE OF THE LUCKY LEGS	Erle Stanley Gardner	2/6
CASE OF THE VELVET CLAWS	Erle Stanley Gardner	2/6
CASE OF THE SULKY GIRL	Erle Stanley Gardner	2/6
RETREAT TO INNOCENCE	Doris Lessing	5/-
ATLAN	Jane Gaskell	5/-
THE CITY	Jane Gaskell	5/-
THE SERPENT	Jane Gaskell	5/-
LIGHT OF THE WESTERN STARS	Zane Grey	3/6
RIDERS OF VENGEANCE	Zane Grey	3/6
THE RAINBOW TRAIL	Zane Grey	3/6
PRAIRIE GOLD	Zane Grey	3/6
DESERT HERITAGE	Zane Grey	3/6

Office: Bookcase 23 Shelf 2.

If you have enjoyed this book and wish to have a complete, free list of Sphere Books, please write to

SPHERE
40 PARK STREET
LONDON W.1.

Sphere Books are available at your bookseller and newsagent. If you wish to order any title from us, please post the full price of the book or books, plus 1/– per book to cover postage and packing, with your order to

SPHERE
40 PARK STREET
LONDON W.1.